1 MINUTE A DAY
TO A
HEALTHIER
YOU

Dr. Bob's

1 MINUTE A DAY TO A
HEALTHIER
YOU

One Minute A Day **Health for a Lifetime**

Dr. Robert DeMaria
THE DRUGLESS DOCTOR

DESTINY IMAGE® PUBLISHERS, INC.

P.O. Box 310, Shippensburg, PA 17257-0310

"Promoting Inspired Lives."

This book and all other Destiny Image, Revival Press, MercyPlace, Fresh Bread, Destiny Image Fiction, and Treasure House books are available at Christian bookstores and distributors worldwide.

For a U.S. bookstore nearest you, call 1-800-722-6774.

For more information on foreign distributors, call 717-532-3040.

Reach us on the Internet: www.destinyimage.com.

ISBN 13 TP: 978-0-7684-0363-3
ISBN 13 Ebook: 978-0-7684-8493-9

For Worldwide Distribution, Printed in the U.S.A.
4 5 6 7 8 / 17 16 15

REFRESHING WATER

*Repent therefore and be converted, that
your sins may be blotted out, so that
times of refreshing may come from the
presence of the Lord....* —ACTS 3:19

Many people do not drink adequate amounts of pure water. Water promotes life. Water bathes the cells and helps eliminate toxins. Take your body weight and divide that number by 4. That number is the minimal number of ounces you should consume.

WATER REFRESHES THE BODY

And the Spirit of God was hovering over the face of the waters. —GENESIS 1:2

Water is essential for life. Water is so essential to life that God refers to water in one of the first Bible verses. Start your day with a cup of hot water and lemon. This is an excellent liver-cleansing stimulant.

YOUR ATTITUDE DETERMINES YOUR ALTITUDE

Your attitude of being proactive about your health should be grounded in the fact that you have a say in what your health future will be. Take the position now to become what you eat, think, and say. Be a blessing and tell someone.

Day 4

HAPPY HEART, CLEAR SKIN

And while [Uzziah] was angry with the priests, leprosy [skin eruptions] broke out on his forehead.... —SECOND CHRONICLES 26:19

Clean machines always work better. When people neglect to drink pure water, they can accumulate toxic backup. An overloaded, toxic liver is the second leading reason people have issues with their skin. Carrots are an excellent source of vitamin A that promote skin and liver health.

Day 5

A WALK BY THE SEA

Again, departing from the region of Tyre and Sidon, He came through the midst of the region of Decapolis to the Sea of Galilee. —MARK 7:31

Walking by a saltwater sea or a fresh body of water is beneficial for body cleansing. Ocean waves can create a negative ion charge. This promotes health and healing. The negative ions pull unwanted toxins from the body via the lymphatic system and literally charge you up. Your body absorbs minerals from the ocean. Take a home mineral bath with Epsom salts to promote health.

WHAT DO I EAT AND DRINK?

Look at the birds of the air, for they neither sow nor reap nor gather into barns; yet your heavenly Father feeds them. Are you not of more value than they? —MATTHEW 6:26

Keep your diet simple and pure. Eat foods that decay and spoil—foods that need to be consumed in a few days. Avoid processed foods. Start your day with one half of a red apple with two teaspoons of organic almond butter, a poached egg, or quinoa. Avoid gluten-based grains like rye, wheat, oats, and barley, as they may be creating health challenges.

Day 7

SO MANY CHOICES

A righteous man who falters before the wicked is like a murky spring and a polluted well. —PROVERBS 25:26

We have many choices when it comes to water. Always check the purity of your water. Spring water may contain high levels of contaminants. Do not drink water that tastes, smells, or looks particulate. Tap water that has an odor of chlorine in the winter months should be avoided. I encourage my patients to drink "reverse osmosis" filtered water.

DRINK WATER ONLY

Wine makes you mean, beer makes you quarrelsome—a staggering drunk is not much fun. —PROVERBS 20:1 THE MESSAGE

Water is essential to promote a quality life. Consuming alcohol creates additional stress on an already overworked liver. Your liver is your recycle organ; keep it pure by drinking pure water.

STOP KIDNEY STONES

Most people who suffer with kidney stones made of calcium oxalate (the most common kind) excrete too much calcium in their urine. A new study has shown that eating less animal protein and using less salt works far better than cutting back on calcium. Limit your daily animal protein to 50 grams or less and your sodium intake to 2,400 milligrams.

Day 10

A Cup of Cold Water

*And whoever gives one of these little ones
only a cup of cold water in the name of a
disciple, assuredly, I say to you, he shall by no
means lose his reward.* —Matthew 10:42

Water purifies the body and is a satisfying thirst quencher. Beware of sugary soft drinks and fruit juices. One twelve-ounce can of soda contains nearly ten teaspoons of sugar. The immune system is paralyzed for hours after eating or drinking sugar. Select grape juice sweetened spritzers as a soda option and herbal tea with fresh mint leaves in place of coffee.

WHAT IS YOUR WATER SOURCE?

Now Jacob's well was there. Jesus therefore,
being wearied from His journey, sat
thus by the well.... —JOHN 4:6

If you have challenging health conditions, test your water sources. Some people believe well water is pure, but herbicides, pesticides, and fertilizers have often contaminated our water tables and wells. Test your drinking water and the water you bathe in.

PROTECT YOURSELF FROM WORLDWIDE POLLUTION

...Because the creation itself also will be delivered from the bondage of corruption in the glorious liberty of the children of God. For we know that the whole creation groans and labors with birth pangs together until now. —ROMANS 8:21-22

We live in a polluted world and creation groans for the return of Jesus so it can be delivered from corruption. Be kind to your liver and drink water from a pure source to cleanse your liver and cleanse your system. Minimize the direct toxins you put into your body.

A Blessed Memory

Blessings are on the head of the righteous.... The memory of the righteous is blessed.... —Proverbs 10:6-7

The brain center for memory is called the hippocampus. It is a major storage center for zinc. Zinc is depleted by wheat, soy, and sugar. Add zinc-rich raw pumpkin seeds to your raw nut salad.

DEAD SEA CLAY

*And Lot lifted his eyes and saw all
the plain of Jordan, that it was well
watered everywhere…like the garden
of the Lord….* —GENESIS 13:10

The Dead Sea contains minerals that can purify and detox your system. Apply Dead Sea mud and clay masks to cleanse your skin of toxins and acne. Alternatively, soak your feet in Epsom salt water to stimulate detoxification.

Day 15

FLUID RETENTION–
DROPSY (KIDNEY
FAILURE)

*And behold, there was a certain man before
Him who had dropsy. ....And He...healed
him, and let him go.* —LUKE 14:2,4

Dropsy—fluid retention, swelling, edema,
and swollen ankles—is the result of a
toxic liver. Increasing protein consumption
can also relieve the body of extra fluid. Avoid
white potatoes, which are a nightshade vegetable and may create water retention. Parsley
is an excellent kidney purifying herb.

Carbonated Beverages and Soft Drinks Increase Body Weight

Weight gain has been linked to the increased consumption of soft drinks and sugary juice drinks. My patients often report headaches, allergies, and high blood pressure when they consume large quantities of sugar. Reduce your risk for diabetes and weight gain by limiting soda consumption to once a month.

Day 17

DRINK LIVING WATER

And the Spirit and the bride say, "Come!" And let him who hears say, "Come!" And let him who thirsts come. Whoever desires, let him take the water of life freely. —REVELATION 22:17

The desire for water is an inborn need required for survival. It is so necessary to our health that Jesus compared the desire for spiritual growth to thirst. Water is not tea, soda, coffee, juice, milk, alcohol, or sports drinks. Water is pure, with nothing added to it. Drink pure water to prevent unhealthy body signals such as constipation, headaches, skin rashes, bad breath, and sinusitis.

Day 18

PAY FOR WATER?

We pay for the water we drink....
—LAMENTATIONS 5:4

Fresh water is a precious commodity. Toxic waste, poor filtration, and chemical neutralizers have limited our access to fresh water. Do not drink unpurified tap water. Most people mistake the craving for water as hunger and eat food when they should actually be drinking more water. Try drinking eight ounces of pure water the next time you feel hungry.

THE LORD USES ORDINARY PEOPLE FOR EXTRAORDINARY ASSIGNMENTS

And Jethro the priest of Midian,
Moses' father-in-law, heard of all that
God had done for Moses and Israel,
His people.... —EXODUS 18:1

I've noticed that extraordinary responsibility and opportunity for achievement were given to individuals with ordinary life experiences. Are you ready for the next level? Replicate what you have gleaned by sharing these tips with family and friends.

OPTIMAL THYROID FUNCTION

*Your teeth are like a flock of sheep which
have come up from the washing....*
—SONG OF SOLOMON 6:6

White teeth are a sign of optimal body function. Are your teeth yellow? Yellow-tinted teeth usually appear with sluggish thyroid function. Cold hands or feet, thinning hair, and a basal body temperature below 97.8 degrees are all signs of poor thyroid function. If you have any of these symptoms, try increasing consumption of supplements like organic kelp, calcium, organic iodine, and flax seeds.

Satisfying Thirst

O God, You are my God; early will I seek
You; my soul thirsts for You; my flesh
longs for You in a dry and thirsty land
where there is no water. —Psalm 63:1

God wants a relationship with us so intently that He relates it to the desire to satisfy thirst. Read the labels on the drinks you consume. Sport drinks do not promote life if they have sugar, high fructose corn syrup, or artificial coloring. Chocolate milk often contains a chemical called theobromine or methyl-xanthine. Drink pure water and herbal tea instead.

Day 22

BETHLEHEM WATER

And David said with longing, "Oh, that someone would give me a drink of the water from the well of Bethlehem, which is by the gate!" —SECOND SAMUEL 23:15

Imagine the sweet taste of water that Jesus consumed at Jacob's well. Who would have thought there would be a point in our lives when we would be searching for pure sources of water? Water with microscopic particles, whether organic from the soil or inorganic from a human-made substance, creates unnecessary stress on our body's very sensitive kidney water filtration system. Avoid water that is not pleasant to the taste—it may contain harmful substances.

BREATH OF LIFE BREAKFAST

Jesus said to them, "Come and eat breakfast...." —JOHN 21:12

Whatever Jesus did is relevant—including that He cooked breakfast for His disciples. The word breakfast means "breaking the fast." Think of your body as a furnace requiring fuel. My suggestion would be to put protein in your machine, which is similar to placing a slow-burning log or coal on a fire. Start every day with a protein or moderate glycemic index breakfast food.

I FREE YOU THIS DAY

*And now look, I free you this day from
the chains that were on your hand. ...
all the land [time] is before you; wherever
it seems good and convenient for you
to go, go there.* —JEREMIAH 40:4

You are free! You are free! Believers in Jesus are free from sin and death! Throw off the shackles of physical and emotional sickness. Follow natural, biblical health principles for optimal health.

TIME FOR BREAKFAST

Jesus...took the bread and gave it to them,
and likewise the fish. —JOHN 21:13

"Come and eat breakfast," Jesus said to Peter after he caught 153 fish. I am sure Jesus was preparing Peter for his massive catch. Fish was a big part of the diet of the Israelites, and fish is a great source of Omega 3 oils. Omega 3 fat supports blood vessels, heart, brain, and nerve health. Add salmon and flax seeds to your diet.

OLD TESTAMENT FOOD

Then God said, "Let the earth bring
forth grass, the herb that yields seed, and
the fruit tree that yields fruit according
to its kind, whose seed is in itself, on the
earth"; and it was so. —GENESIS 1:11

One of the main obstacles to a healthy diet is knowing what to eat. Old Testament food was not genetically altered to resist pests. Avoid mutated or seedless vegetables and fruit. Focus on organic, non-genetically modified food.

Day 27

GAS PEDAL

While the earth remains, seedtime and harvest, cold and heat, winter and summer, and day and night shall not cease. —GENESIS 8:22

Imagine your body is like a machine. The liver is the oil filter, the lungs are the muffler, the brain is the electric circuit, and your thyroid is the gas pedal. The thyroid helps the body adjust to hot and cold. If the initial cold of winter penetrates your bones, you may need more iodine in your diet. Add iodine-rich foods like Celtic Sea Salt, organic kelp, and sea vegetables to your diet.

Day 28

ABUNDANT FRUIT

*Like an apple tree among the trees of
the woods, so is my beloved among the
sons. I sat down in his shade with great
delight, and his fruit was sweet to my
taste.* —SONG OF SOLOMON 2:3

Eat fresh, organic vegetables and fruits.
They are a great source of fiber and are
necessary to cleanse the colon. You can also
lower cholesterol by eating fiber because it
gently scrapes and brushes the mineral-
absorbing intestinal villi. Think "living
food" versus canned, frozen, or commercially prepared, vacuumed food and drink.

FRESH SOURCES OF FIBER

Like an apple tree among the trees of the woods, so is my beloved among the sons. I sat down in his shade with great delight, and his fruit was sweet to my taste. —SONG OF SOLOMON 2:3

Drink fresh, whole juice with nothing artificial added. I suggest investing in a durable juicer to make fresh juice daily. Try drinking eight ounces of fresh juice from organic beets, carrots, celery, apples, parsley, cucumbers, and ginger. Avoid drinking any carton or canned juices that have been pasteurized or concentrated.

THE BEST DIET

People who eat a healthy diet have a 10 to 20 percent lower risk of disease. Take steps toward eating a healthy diet today. Eat five servings of vegetables and four servings of fruit every day. Replace unhealthy snacks with a serving of nuts. Consume more poultry and fish than red meat.

You Are Known by Your Fruit

...Every good tree bears good fruit, but a bad tree bears bad fruit. A good tree cannot bear bad fruit, nor can a bad tree bear good fruit. —MATTHEW 7:17-18

Healthy people are happy people. Fruit consumption restores important nutrients in the body. Fruit is a great source of fiber, especially the apple, which is necessary to keep your bowels functioning regularly. An apple a day keeps the doctor away!

DR. BOB'S ABCs FOR LIFE

He causes...vegetation for the service of man.... —PSALM 104:14

There were fruit trees, plants, and herbs to sustain life in the Garden of Eden. Eat your ABCs in fruit. Apples have malic acid to help thin bile for better digestion. Beets are full of fiber that cleanses the intestinal wall. Carrots have vitamin A that support skin, eye, and liver health.

YOGURT—GOOD OR BAD?

All things are lawful for me, but not all things are helpful; all things are lawful for me, but not all things edify.
—FIRST CORINTHIANS 10:23

Paul said all things are lawful for us but not necessarily good for us. Commercial, conventional American yogurt has permeated the breakfast and snack market. Yogurt is a great source of protein, but read the labels and brands with sugar and high fructose corn syrup. Sprinkle sesame seeds on your favorite dish for a boost of calcium.

A PINK TOOTHBRUSH

Americans get a limited amount of natural vitamin C complex from their diet. Lack of vitamin C can create weakness in teeth and gums resulting in fragile gum tissue and a pink toothbrush. Avoid eating synthetic vitamin C tablets; the acid is tough on the enamel. Eat bell peppers, which are an excellent source of complex C.

SWINE, GO SWIMMING

Now a large herd of swine was feeding there near the mountains. ...Then [with Jesus' permission] *the unclean spirits went out and entered the swine...and the herd ran violently down the steep place into the sea, and drowned in the sea.* —MARK 5:11,13

Swine were and still are unclean animals. Pork is not the other white meat. Pork flesh, no matter how you cook it, is toxic. Do you have a relentless thirst after eating ham or bacon? Your body is attempting to dilute toxins. Pass on the pork and try turkey bacon.

WHAT SHALL WE EAT?

*...For your heavenly Father knows that you
need all these things.* —MATTHEW 6:32

Food is an integral part of God's Word.
Your body is required to work harder
and can become stressed as it attempts to
keep you functioning on dead, devitalized
food. The pancreas is especially stressed by
providing enzymes to properly break down
"fake" food. Eat living food, food without
labels. Avoid all processed items.

VITAMIN E AND YOUR EYES

Vitamin E supports eye health. Supplements have not been proven to reduce the risk of macular degeneration. Your safest bet is to eat a diet rich in fruits, vegetables, and leafy greens.

Day 38

PURE SALT

Your body needs sodium. Sodium is an important mineral needed to reduce body stiffness and control allergies. But sodium chloride or "table salt" is an unhealthy combination. Use Celtic Sea Salt. Celtic Sea Salt is pure and not whitened or chemically altered.

AN EGG A DAY

Eggs are one of the most complete foods on the planet, but we have lived in "egg phobia" for nearly thirty years. Eggs are an excellent source of protein. Egg yolk has lecithin in it, which helps emulsify the cholesterol. Eat free range, organic eggs. Stay away from "plastic" liquid eggs in a carton.

MELONS—FRUIT OF THE VINE

We remember the fish which we ate freely in Egypt, the cucumbers, the melons.... —NUMBERS 11:5

God created an inborn desire for sweets for survival. Human milk has a natural sweetness, but creating a sugar addiction in your infants and toddlers can cause a lifetime of health issues. Limit your consumption of high sugar fruits like watermelon. Substitute a wedge of cucumber, a relative to the watermelon, for your potassium instead of a high-carbohydrate banana.

Day 41

A WHIP FOR A HORSE

Do not fear therefore; you are of more value than many sparrows. —MATTHEW 10:31

What do you feed your body? Are you not more important than the sparrow? Feed your body whole food. Avoid deli meats; eat baked fries versus oil-cooked; treat yourself to quality ice cream; pass on the hot dogs. Start your day with food for a champion athlete: an egg and wholesome, fresh, organic almond butter on sprouted grain bread.

BRING TO REMEMBRANCE

...He [the Holy Spirit] *will teach you all things, and bring to your remembrance all things that I said to you.* —JOHN 14:26

God created our memory as a human secret weapon. You can increase your memory capacity by detoxifying your body. A poor diet can stress the liver, the cleansing organ for the body. Critical brain food for memory health is eating Omega 3 fat from plant sources. Add some flax seeds to your whole grain cereal in the morning.

BLUEBERRIES AND ANTIOXIDANTS

*...For why is my liberty judged
by another man's conscience?* —
FIRST CORINTHIANS 10:29

Focus your daily activity to limit obvious damage from pollutants and toxins. While working at home or in the yard, it is prudent to follow directions to keep skin, lungs, and clothing from being exposed to hazardous chemicals. You can promote cellular health and protection by choosing foods that act as natural barriers to toxins similar to a clear coat of wax on motor vehicles. Blueberries are a great source of antioxidants and promote cellular repair.

Day 44

DR. BOB'S BREAKFAST

Jesus said to them, "Come and eat breakfast." —JOHN 21:12

What is the breakfast of champions? Focus on medium or low glycemic index foods for breakfast, like protein. Avoid foods that elevate insulin, like breakfast cereals. Try starting your day with scrambled eggs and spinach. If you do eat bread, add almond butter or olive oil instead of butter and jam. If you like oatmeal, add flax seeds, almonds, or shredded coconut for healthy oils.

FRUIT AND VEGGIE DIET

Those who boosted their intake of fruits and vegetables by four servings a day had a 24 percent lower risk of obesity than those who cut their fruits and vegetables by about two servings a day. Pack some baby carrots for snacks, start breakfast with wedges of cantaloupe, and serve at least two vegetables for dinner. Who can complain about roasted asparagus, broccoli in garlic sauce, or sautéed spinach?

NIGHTSHADE VEGETABLES

B e aware that the nightshade food group may create pain and distress in your body. Nightshade vegetables include tomatoes, white potatoes, green peppers, hot peppers, eggplant, and paprika. Nightshade vegetables compromise liver function. Rebuild your liver by avoiding these stressful vegetables.

EXERCISE FOR LIFE

Regular exercise promotes efficient burning of blood sugar. Muscles need fuel to perform their purpose. You can help control your blood glucose by simple activities, including walking, bike riding, and jogging. Choose a regular activity with motion. Ships in the harbor attract rust and barnacles. Don't go down with the ship! Keep moving!

Day 48

WALK YOUR WAY TO HEALTH

*And everyone who competes for the
prize is temperate in all things. Now
they do it to obtain a perishable crown,
but we for an imperishable crown.*
—FIRST CORINTHIANS 9:25

Experts suggest that walking ten thousand steps daily, or about five miles, will help burn off some extra calories you have consumed. Each mile is about 2,500 steps. It takes 7,990 steps to burn off the average cheeseburger. Doughnuts take 5,750 steps; a 12-ounce can of soda takes 3,450 steps; a garden salad with fat-free dressing takes 1,160 steps.

BUILDING MUSCLE STRENGTH

...And works it with the strength of his arms.... —ISAIAH 44:12

As we mature, we lose muscle firmness and strength. A poor metabolism can result in a zinc deficiency. Low zinc levels reduce insulin output, and your body needs fuel in the cells through by insulin. Reduce refined carbs and start light to moderate muscle strengthening to promote solid bone integrity.

OBESITY EPIDEMIC

My people are destroyed for lack of
knowledge.... —HOSEA 4:6

Manufacturers are required by law to list product ingredients. To reach your goal of optimal health, you must obtain nutrition knowledge and become a label reader. Don't be ignorant of the facts. Avoid food with high fructose corn syrup, which prevents your stomach from recognizing it is full.

CRAVINGS

*And the world passes away and disappears,
and with it the forbidden cravings....*
—FIRST JOHN 2:17 AMPLIFIED BIBLE

Increase your protein consumption during the day to reduce cravings for sugar and carbohydrates. This will also help to reduce blood pressure. Sugar robs the body of minerals and vitamins. If you crave sugar, wean yourself off sugar by increasing consumption of low fat proteins.

CORNERSTONE SIGNIFICANCE

Having been built on the foundation of the apostles and prophets, Jesus Christ Himself being the chief cornerstone. —EPHESIANS 2:20

The cornerstone in your body frame is the spine. For optimal health, we need to focus on standing and sitting erect. Here is a tip. When standing, focus on holding your shoulders back. Grasp your hands and place them in the small of your back. This will naturally position your shoulders behind a forward head alignment. Spinal breakdown is effortless—erect posture requires energy.

Day 53

SUNNING

...Because the sun has tanned me....
—SONG OF SOLOMON 1:6

God put the sun in the sky to provide light for up to sixteen hours a day. The sun's rays are part of a health wellness plan. Sunlight converts the cholesterol in your skin to vitamin D, which is needed for calcium absorption. Cold sores can be caused by a lack of calcium in your diet. Consume additional flax seed oil and calcium citrate when you know you will be in the sun more than usual.

Day 54

STAND TALL

*Put on the whole armor of God, that
you may be able to stand against the
wiles of the devil.* —EPHESIANS 6:11

Look at your posture; others do. Is your
trunk in a forward position? Are your
shoulders round? The "Doorjamb Push-Up"
will help stabilize your trunk position and
vitalize your lung capacity. Stand in the
middle of a doorway. Raise your hands to
shoulder height or above, place the palms
on the doorjamb, and lean your body into
the doorway. Remain in the position for five
seconds. Do this exercise daily—three sets
of fifteen.

STAND FOR TRUTH

Stand therefore, having girded your waist with truth, having put on the breastplate of righteousness. —EPHESIANS 6:14

A forward head position is one of the most challenging to slow, stop, and reverse. Lay down on a weight bench, picnic table bench, or a coffee table. While lying on your back, slide your head/trunk to the end of your support structure. Slide off until you are mid-shoulder blade or lower. Hang your head, shoulders, and upper trunk off the edge for thirty seconds. This is an excellent active maneuver, which strengthens the trunk and pulls the upper body backward.

STAND AGAINST EVIL

*Therefore take up the whole armor of
God, that you may be able to withstand
in the evil day, and having done all,
to stand.* —EPHESIANS 6:13

An optimal functioning spine means an optimal functioning nervous system, and you can slow the destructive compression of gravity with the following exercise. Sit in a chair with your eyes closed. Slide your head and upper neck straight backward, then tilt chin up slightly. Do not move your shoulders. Hold the position for five seconds. This is an excellent way to establish and maintain a normal cervical curve.

MENTAL CONTENTMENT

*Not that I speak in regard to need, for
I have learned in whatever state I am,
to be content.* —PHILIPPIANS 4:11

Mental confusion, mental instability, or noises in the head can be a sign of whole food B vitamin deficiency. Having constant noises and emotional turmoil can create chaos and drain you emotionally. Self-inflicted negative self-talk can also deplete necessary B vitamins. Sugar is by far the leading cause of B vitamin deficiency. Add whole-grain B vitamin food to your meals like oats, rye, millet, spelt, barley, and brown rice.

A BIT OF HISTORY— STEP CLIMBING

Then they led Jesus from Caiaphas to the Praetorium, and it was early morning. ... Pilate then when out to them.... —JOHN 18:28

Stair climbing is an excellent cardio-vascular exercise for your heart and lungs. I encourage my patients to walk regularly. A stair-step machine is a valu-able piece of equipment that strengthens your butt muscles and supports your spine and thigh muscles and will even tighten up painful weak knees. Walk up the steps instead of using the escalator or elevator. You will reduce pain and improve back and knee strength.

KNOWLEDGE AND PASSION

For God so loved the world that He gave His only begotten Son.... —JOHN 3:16

The food you eat becomes you. Hot dogs, bologna, fries, and soda become your nerves, eyes, hair, blood, and emotional state. Regular exercise diminishes depression without the need for medications. Sugar fogs the mind and memory. Lack of sleep slows sharpness in decisions. Exercise, by far, is the one activity that will do a lot for increasing your energy and mental acuity.

DIABETES: ZERO RISK

Women who engage in at least seven hours a week of brisk walking, heavy gardening, or housework vigorous enough to build up a sweat have a 30 percent lower risk of diabetes than women who exercise less than half an hour a week. Women who eat high-fiber cereals and breads (rather than sweets, potatoes, and other refined carbohydrates) reduce their risk of diabetes by half.

STEPS TO RESTORE HEALTH

For I will restore health to you.... —JEREMIAH 30:17

Focus on living food versus processed, overcooked, and chemically altered "wannabe" foods. Clean machines work better—drink water from a pure source. Begin a regular "oxygen stimulating" exercise routine such as aerobics, walking, or weight training. Exercise keeps the frame toned and solid. Sleep a minimum of six to eight hours nightly. Getting to sleep before midnight is life enhancing. You do not want to depend on your "second wind"—your immune system will be stressed.

FOOT GEAR

And he preached, saying, "There comes One after me who is mightier than I, whose sandal strap I am not worthy to stoop down and loose." —MARK 1:7

If you daily spend a full eight to ten hours on your feet—change your shoes halfway through the day. Your feet will thank you. I regularly change shoes since I am on my feet for extended periods of time. Dress for comfort. Shoes that are old and worn out should be replaced.

JOHN AND PETER RAN

*So they both ran together, and the
other disciple outran Peter and came
to the tomb first.* —JOHN 20:4

Running, jogging, and fast walking helps burn extra calories. Find an exercise partner and stay fit. My wife, Deb, and I run every morning beginning at 5:45 a.m. Running together gives us an opportunity to share twenty minutes of uninterrupted conversation, and it helps us keep our calories under control and in balance.

ENERGIZE ME!

*And we desire that each one of you show
the same diligence to the full assurance of
hope to the end, that you do not become
sluggish....* —HEBREWS 6:11-12

A common dilemma in our laser-lane society is lack of energy. There are many possible reasons for no get-up-and-go. A very common one is that your body does not have enough zinc. Avoid zinc-depleting foods like sugar, wheat, and soy; your body will restore its own reserve of zinc. Low zinc levels may create large facial pores, slow healing time, memory lapses, prostrate swelling, and excessive scar or keloid formation.

RESTORING FUNCTION

*…"Let us rise up and build." Then
they set their hands to this good
work.* —NEHEMIAH 2:18

Clean machines work better. Add measured amounts of pure water to your daily protocol. Your appetite pattern will stabilize, skin integrity will improve, bowels will be consistent, and pain will disappear. Seek food that is organic, fresh, and locally grown. Focus on vegetables, whole grains, and lean meat; avoid wheat and dairy. Do not end meals with fruit.

PHYSICALLY FIT, KINGDOM FIT

But Jesus said to him, "No one, having put his hand to the plow, and looking back, is fit for the kingdom of God." —LUKE 9:62

Choose to be around people who are pro-active self-starters. When you start down the road to optimal health and continue to pursue a healthier you, you will discover how gratified and motivated you become. Do not look back.

DUCKING DIABETES

Get off the couch, office chair, or driver's seat for at least twenty to thirty minutes of walking or other activity every day. Cut calories with a healthy diet that includes lots of fruits and vegetables. Don't miss meals. Use lunch time as a time to refuel in the middle of the day. Your blood sugar does not need a blast of empty fast food or convenience calories. Try a mixed green salad with protein,

"HOLD THE PICKLE"

*And the Daughter of Zion...is left like
a...booth in a vineyard, like a lodge in
a garden of cucumbers, like a besieged
city....* —ISAIAH 1:8 AMPLIFIED BIBLE

Eat cucumbers as a source of potassium instead of bananas. Bananas tend to constipate and contain a lot of sugar. Be aware of pickled cucumbers; they can irritate your liver. Do not eat a lot of sweet pickles! Cucumbers, Celtic Sea Salt, onions, and organic sour cream make a delightful salad. Sprinkle dill seed on raw cucumbers for a zesty snack!

PASS THE MUSTARD

The Kingdom of Heaven is like a mustard seed planted in a field. It is the smallest of all seeds, but it becomes the largest of garden plants; it grows into a tree, and birds come and make nests in its branches. —MATTHEW 13:31-32 NEW LIVING TRANSLATION

Prior to modern pain relieving medication, mustard, in the form of mustard plaster or mustard paper, was used as a treatment for rheumatism. Some spice mixes have turmeric in them. Turmeric is also a natural pain reliever. It prevents the formation of a pain producing tissue-like-hormone called Prostaglandin 2. Omit the pain-producing hydrogenated fat in mayonnaise and instead add extra mustard.

RUSTPROOF YOURSELF

*...where neither moth nor rust nor
worm consume and destroy....* —
MATTHEW 6:20 AMPLIFIED BIBLE

Antioxidants are a vital part of our diet because they slow down the process of bodily decay. Blueberries are by far one of the best antioxidants. Fresh greens like spinach also act as "rustproofers." The more servings of fresh veggies and fruit you eat, the better protected you are against "rust." Fresh or self-frozen blueberries are an excellent year-round source of antioxidants.

WINNING THE PAIN GAME

...much pain is in every side.... —NAHUM 2:10

Insidious, or chronic pain (the annoying type), can literally wear a person out. Sugar, nightshade vegetables, and cow's milk can contribute to chronic pain. Fat can relieve your aches and discomfort. Take one tablespoon of organic flax seed oil per 100 pounds of body weight. This promotes PG3, a pain-relieving prostaglandin.

Day 72

A STRONG VOICE

Your watchmen shall lift up their voices, with their voices they shall sing together.... —ISAIAH 52:8

Many people struggle with issues in their vocal region. Stress can aggravate these issues. The vocal cord region can also be congested due to a sulfur deficiency. Sulfur is needed to thin phlegm and drainage and is needed for fat metabolism. Grate a sulfur-rich egg on your mixed green lunch salad. Add potassium-rich cucumber slices to your meal.

Day 73

NUT BUTTER

*So their father, Jacob, finally said to them,
"If it can't be avoided, then at least do this.
Pack your bags with the best products of
this land. Take them down to the man as
gifts*—BALM, HONEY, GUM, AROMATIC
RESIN, PISTACHIO *nuts, and almonds.* —
Genesis 43:11 New Living Translation

Do you suffer from chronic sinus pain?
Peanuts and peanut butter may be the
main reason for your sinus pain and chronic
dripping nose. Peanuts are not actually nuts;
they are legumes and are considered to be in
the nightshade family, a family of plants that
contain poisonous juice. Try eating almond
or cashew butter.

GOOD FOR THE HEART

People who eat beans, almond butter, and other legumes at least four times a week have a 29 percent lower risk of heart disease than those who eat legumes less than once a week. Eat more beans. Think of them not as beans, but as chick pea curry, split pea soup, rice and lentils, burritos, hummus, and Pasta e Fagioli.

DETOXIFICATION

Purge [cleanse] *me with hyssop, and I shall be clean; wash me, and I shall be whiter than snow.* —PSALM 51:7

We live in a very toxic environment. Detoxifying starts by stopping. You need to stop consuming processed food, human-made oils, sugar, and artificial colors. We are exposed to toxins through lawn applications, oven cleaners, home pesticides, paint cleaners, vehicle exhaust, and so forth. Even in a relatively clean environment, our cells accumulate waste products as part of normal living. Add raw, organic beets to your salad to help your liver get cleansed.

Day 76

FOOD FOR THOUGHT

So He humbled you, allowed you to hunger, and fed you with manna which you did not know nor did your fathers know, that He might make you know that man shall not live by bread alone; but man lives by every word that proceeds from the mouth of the Lord. —DEUTERONOMY 8:3

What should you eat to think clearly? The brain is made of fat. Eating the right fat or nutrients to make brain fat promotes brain health. Eat Omega 3 fats like those in flax seed oil. Rather than smearing butter or margarine on bread, substitute those spreads for flax or olive oil. Your brain will thank you!

Day 77

WHAT ABOUT CHEESE?

*And carry these ten cheeses to the captain
of their thousand, and see how your
brothers fare, and bring back news
of them.* —FIRST SAMUEL 17:18

Goat cheese was a common staple of the biblical diet. In biblical times, heat or chemicals did not alter the process of fermentation and enzyme action in cheese making like it does today. Cheese is a logical way to incorporate dairy into your life, but many people cannot tolerate much dairy without experiencing mild pain or sinus issues. Focus on raw, organic cheese without additives. Do not eat human-made cheese in a can, box, or with colors or additives.

BLIND AS A BAT

*And the men who journeyed with
him stood speechless, hearing a voice
but seeing no one.* —ACTS 9:7

Your eyesight is affected by the nutrients you eat. Eyes require an excellent blood supply and vitamin A. Challenges of night vision impairment can improve by eating a quality source of organic carrots. Fresh, raw carrots are best. Floaters in your eyes diminish with vitamin A and liver cleansing. The liver uses and stores vitamin A. When the liver is short on vitamin A, it "borrows" it from the eyes. Try freshly squeezed carrot juice for a boost of vitamin A.

GIVE US OUR DAILY BREAD

Give us this day our daily bread. —MATTHEW 6:11

I have seen chronic allergies eliminated by ceasing to eat wheat products. The protein in wheat, called gluten, can create an "alarm attack" in the body. Headaches, body pain, sinusitis, digestive distress, and even tremors can be a reaction to wheat. Test yourself and go without wheat for a month. Try spelt grain bread instead of wheat bread. Limit your bread consumption.

CURDS FROM CATTLE

Did You not pour me out like milk, and curdle me like cheese. —JOB 10:10

Dairy items such as milk, cottage cheese, and ice cream can be the primary cause of chronic pain. You need to be a label reader and study the ingredients in any dairy product you ingest. Thousands of people thrive without dairy in their diet, contrary to popular belief. Conventionally raised cattle are medicated with antibiotics, growth hormones, and steroids. Focus on organic dairy items.

SALAD SAVVY

Will you walk away from the table with fewer calories if you start your meal with a salad? It depends on the salad!

Start dinner with a salad that is mostly vegetables. Avoid calorie-dense salad dressings. If you aren't a fan of fat-free dressing, try organic reduced-fat (as little as possible) and skip the cheese, croutons, Chinese noodles, and other calorie-dense salad trimmings like bacon bits.

ACCELERATED HEALING

But He was wounded for our transgressions,
He was bruised for our guilt and iniquities....
—ISAIAH 53:5 AMPLIFIED BIBLE

Are you bruising easily and without cause? Eat more greens and bell peppers. Greens are an excellent source of chlorophyll, which promote vitamin K utilization. Lack of vitamin C can also result in bruising. Red, orange, and yellow bell peppers are great sources of vitamin C. Slow healers with excess scarring normally have low zinc and high copper. Eat a plant-rich diet to promote health.

PREVENT PESTILENCE

Nor of the pestilence that walks in darkness, nor of the destruction that lays waste at noonday. —PSALM 91:6

Pestilence can be any event or condition, internal or external, that interferes with your ability to thrive as God intended. A modern-day pestilence is cancer. I applaud the progress that has been achieved so far, but is irradiating and injecting chemicals into a body with a stressed immune system the logical approach? Clean machines work the best. Avoid foods that are fried. Eat fresh, organic produce.

SANDWICHES

…"Where could we get enough bread in the wilderness to fill such a great multitude?" —MATTHEW 15:33

Are you thirsty after a meal? Your body is attempting to dilute the poison you just consumed. Combining protein (meat requiring acid to digest) along with carbohydrates (bread requiring alkalinity) confuses the system. Loading up veggies between whole grain bread is a safe option. Do you want deli meat? Buy an organic variety that does not contain hormones or preservatives. Roll up a slice with your favorite veggies or lettuce, and chew it thoroughly. Your stomach will thank you.

PEPPERMINT LEAVES

*Woe to you, scribes and Pharisees, pretenders
(hypocrites)! For you give a tenth of your mint
and dill and cumin and have neglected and
omitted the weightier...matters of the Law....*
—MATTHEW 23:23 AMPLIFIED BIBLE

There must have been some value to mint in the New Testament since Jesus made mention of it in regard to the Pharisees paying a tithe on it. The exact variety is not mentioned, but all mints are very aromatic. Mint is very stimulating to the palate—it will put a little spring in your step. The essential oil obtained from mint leaves contains menthol, which is used as a cooling remedy. Add peppermint leaves to your favorite herbal tea.

Skip the Milk

*For everyone who partakes only of milk is
unskilled in the word of righteousness, for he
is a babe. But solid food belongs to those who
are of full age, that is, those who by reason
of use have their senses exercised to discern
both good and evil.* —Hebrews 5:13-14

Substances derived from cow's milk are more difficult to digest. Protein in milk can create chronic allergies. Cow's milk has more calcium for cow bones and less phospholipids for brains. The million dollar question: Where do cows get their calcium? Ice cream, cheese, yogurt, or milk? No! They eat hay, grass, and alfalfa. Now I don't want you to go out and graze in the field, but eating living food does make sense.

DR. BOB'S LUNCH

*And Jesus took the loaves, and when He
had given thanks He distributed them
to the disciples, and the disciples to those
sitting down; and likewise the fish, as
much as they wanted.* —JOHN 6:11

Consuming a carbohydrate meal without protein for lunch creates a desire for sweets for your midday fueling around 3:00 p.m. Protein is like a slow burning log keeping the machine working steady as she goes. I eat a mixed green (no iceberg) salad that includes radishes, tomatoes, cucumbers, beets, sesame and sunflower seeds, cauliflower, broccoli, cabbage, carrots, parsley, chives, or basil. I use flax oil and beet juice for my dressing. This is a midday fuel for champions!

REFUELING AT LUNCH

Your goal is to eat a light meal in the midday. Adding fruit or dessert on a layer of protein and starches creates the potential for digestive distress. Drink water with lemon or herbal tea. Avoid drinking coffee or soda; caffeinated or highly sugared beverages add stress to your liver.

HIDDEN PAIN TRIGGERS

Gluten may be a stealth cause of a variety of health challenges, including headaches, pain, dark circles under your eyes, digestive distress, and many more. Gluten is a protein found in these commonly used grains: wheat, rye, oats, and barley. If you have chronic health challenges, you may consider going gluten-free for a month.

Day 90

DEADLY NIGHTSHADES

If going gluten-free does not give you pain relief or if other chronic health challenges continue to linger, you want to consider going on a nightshade-free lifestyle for four to six weeks: no tomatoes, white potatoes, green peppers, hot peppers, eggplant, peanuts, or paprika. This regime may seem a bit demanding, but I have learned from experience that pain has everything to do with what you are putting in and on your body.

Day 91

EATING SMART

Foods properly combined streamline digestion, promote weight loss, and energize and strengthen your entire body. What you eat, when you eat, and with whom you eat has an influence on the final product that enters the cell. Eat fruit by itself on an empty stomach. Let twenty to thirty minutes elapse after eating fruit before eating other foods. Animal protein mixes best with non-starch food like broccoli, cabbage, beans, and mixed greens. Avoid pastas, grain, and potatoes with animal protein.

FOOD COMBINATIONS

*The he [Noah] drank of the wine and
was drunk, and became uncovered
in his tent.* —GENESIS 9:21

Eat fruit alone and in the morning, followed by nuts. The nuts limit insulin release. I strongly suggest eliminating fruits after a meal. Eating fruit after a meal results in slowed or delayed indigestion and fermentation. Fermentation of undigested food in a warm, dark environment (your stomach) produces poison gases, foul-smelling stools, and if the combination is right, even alcohol. Eat fruit alone in the morning.

YOU ARE WHAT YOU EAT, DIGEST, ABSORB

...the priest's servant would come with a three-pronged fleshhook in his hand while the meat was boiling. —FIRST SAMUEL 2:13

Digestive distress prevents your body from gathering the nutrients you need to have optimal health. Correct food choices are critical. Avoid processed, devitalized food.

Cooking methods affect the quality of the end product. Boiling draws the minerals and vitamins out of the fiber into the water and down the drain. Raw, lightly steamed, or blanched veggies go a long way in providing your digestive system enzymes for assimilation.

Day 94

YOU ARE THE SALT OF THE EARTH

You are salt of the earth, but if salt has lost its taste…how can its saltiness be restored?
—MATTHEW 5:13 AMPLIFIED BIBLE

Salt is one of those minerals that is misunderstood. Sodium is a mineral. Your body needs minerals. Craving salt is often a sign of weak adrenal function. Adrenal glands make hormones in the body including cortisone. You need real, quality salt! Liberally use Celtic Sea Salt. You can find this product in most health food stores.

Day 95

SHOULDER PAIN

*The God of this people Israel chose our fathers, and exalted the people when they dwelt as strangers in the land of Egypt, and **with an uplifted arm** He brought them out of it.* —ACTS 13:17

Can you raise your arms above your head without pain? There is a common condition that affects the tissues around the muscles and bones of the shoulder called bursitis. Bursitis is often associated with an alkaline saliva pH.

B6 supplementation, along with organic apple cider vinegar, may be needed for a season. Do not drink fluids with your meals. This tends to raise saliva pH.

LEMON ZEST

*And you shall take for yourselves on
the first day the fruit of beautiful
trees....* —LEVITICUS 23:40

According to rabbis, the fruit of "goodly trees" means lemons. Drinking one lemon wedge in eight ounces of hot water every fifteen minutes can either minimize the pain or cause stones to pass naturally. A simple snoring remedy is to drink hot water with a wedge of lemon juice added and then eat the lemon right before bed. Try a cup of water with a fresh lemon wedge, stevia (an herb to sweeten), and mint leaves as a beverage.

COOKING TIPS

*If your grain offering is prepared on a griddle,
it is to be made of the finest flour mixed
with oil, and without yeast.* —LEVITICUS
2:5 NEW INTERNATIONAL VERSION

The poorest nutritional method of cooking food is boiling. The quality of water is significant, and the length of time the item is heated affects the content and value of nutrients left. Boiling draws the nutrient into the water and then the water (and nutrient) is poured down the drain. Baked sweet potatoes and yams are more nutritious than boiled and mashed. The least amount of heat applied to your meal, the more usable nutrients are available for cell restoration.

HEAT DESTROYS NUTRIENTS

Always have raw veggies with a meal providing enzymes that give your pancreas a breather. You can spray olive, high oleic safflower, or sunflower oils from a manual pump sprayer instead of commercially produced hydrogenated "low cholesterol" products. Butter can also be used as a source of frying fat.

Cooking Techniques

So what type of pots and pans do you use to cook? We use stainless steel Cuisinart® cookware. We also bake frequently in our oven using baking bags, which prevent loss of nutrients and reduce cooking time. I bake beets every week, and I also consistently bake chicken and turkey in the oven. As a side note, in my experience, I have not noticed an elevation in hair analysis aluminum levels in individuals who use aluminum cookware.

THE MEDITERRANEAN DIET

Want to stick around to see your great-grandchildren? Eat a healthy Mediterranean diet, exercise, don't smoke, and drink alcohol moderately. Eat less meat, dairy, and saturated fat and more fruits, vegetables, beans, fish, grains, nuts, and unsaturated fats. Don't smoke and stay physically active.

THE NEW RECIPE BOX

Health conditions are not all necessarily genetically passed on. You are what you eat. Ask happy, healthy-looking people what they eat. Copy their recipes. Change what's in your recipe box if your traditional family meals perpetuate poor health. Heavy, rich ethnic foods promote liver stress.

Day 102

HERBS ARE A BLESSING

*For the earth which drinks in the rain that
often comes upon it, and bears **herbs** useful
for those by whom it is cultivated, receives
blessing from God.* —HEBREWS 6:7

Our heavenly Father has provided food and
drink from the beginning. Herbs have
been part of that plan since Genesis. There
are many classifications of herbs. Herbs have
been used to tone, excite, and relax the body
and mind. I have several planting boxes on
my deck at home where I grow herbs. In the
springtime, shop at a greenhouse nursery or
health food store for organic herbs plants
or seeds. This is when you will have the
best selection.

Day 103

HERBS, HERBS, HERBS

Parsley has many varieties. It is an excellent kidney purifier. I suggest, especially with individuals with kidney stress, to eat parsley on their mixed green salads or steep it in hot water and drink it as a tea. Chives add the essence of onion. They are great in scrambled eggs, salads, macaroni, and potato dishes. Dill adds an exciting zest to food. Sage and rosemary are very bold—only use a pinch. Thyme and oregano are awesome in tomato sauce. We snip basil with kitchen shears. It's tasty with thin tomato slices and olive oil.

Day 104

CHICKEN SOUP FOR THE SOUL

As fire burns brushwood, as fire causes water to boil.... —ISAIAH 64:2

Real chicken soup starts with fresh organic chicken, especially thighs and legs. There are natural ingredients in animal protein that stimulate the immune system. Start with quality water, filtered with reverse osmosis. The only time you want to boil anything is when making soups. Use fresh, organic ingredients to enhance the results of your cooking effort. Use rice noodles instead of wheat noodles.

PROPER PH

Like one who takes away a garment in cold weather, and like vinegar [acid] *on soda* [alkalinity]…. —PROVERBS 25:20

Monitoring the pH level in your saliva is a noninvasive tool we use to "check the battery" and determine how the body is functioning. Fruits and vegetables shift the body toward an alkaline state. Meat, grains, and stress tilt it toward the acid side. Acid pH is found in patients who are stressed, eat meat, drink little water, and may have degenerative health problems, even cancer.

TASTE THE WONDERFUL STUFF

Every man at the beginning sets out the good wine, and when the guests have well drunk, then the inferior. You have kept the good wine until now! —JOHN 2:10

Make your own food when asked to bring a dish to an event. Fresh and organic is the secret weapon. Commercially preserved or packaged food is bland and limp. Add your favorite fresh herb or herbs to your salad, entrees, or side dishes instead of commercial taste enhancers. Create simple touches with meals. You will reap the benefit of knowing you shared quality food for a meal. Live it up!

ADDING SPECIAL TOUCHES

Mushrooms sliced thin hold their essence versus mushrooms from a can. Pine nuts, sesame seeds, or walnuts added to a salad or vegetable enhance the protein content and taste. Celery hearts are milder than outer sticks. Lightly grate the peel of lemon for a special accent. Almond or vanilla extract blended with maple syrup over sweet potatoes and/or apples will bring people back for more.

NATURAL FLAVOR SPICES

Five hundred shekels of cassia [cinnamon]…
and a hin of olive oil. —EXODUS 30:24

When God created the planet, He provided for us naturally all of our wants, needs, and desires. One of my favorite spices is cinnamon. The aroma of cinnamon on anything activates every smell and taste receptor in my body. There are many ways to use organic cinnamon. Be creative. Start your day with fresh, gluten-free quinoa or short grain brown rice. Add some raw almonds and a sprinkle of cinnamon.

A HEALTHY DESSERT

Bake some apples (leave the peel on to prevent loss of moisture and nutrients) and sprinkle some cinnamon on them when fork-tender. We make our own applesauce. It's easy. Peel, core, cut the apples into small cubes, and add a small amount of pure water to a cooking pot. Simmer on low heat until tender, smash, and cool. Sprinkle with cinnamon for flavor. Try cinnamon on brown rice or grits. For extraordinary essence, adding cinnamon to oils is a treat. Use some creative imagination.

THE BEST MEDS

Those who eat a healthy Mediterranean diet have less inflammation and insulin resistance. Eat more fruits, vegetables, beans, whole grains, and seafood. Replace saturated fats from meat and dairy with unsaturated fats from oils and nuts.

BEET ROOT

I will be like the dew to Israel; he shall grow like the lily, and lengthen his roots like Lebanon. —HOSEA 14:5

The best way to incorporate organic beets is grated, raw on a mixed green salad. I encourage patients to eat them raw or baked. You can also cut and peel the beets to the size you would cut potatoes to be mashed. Add balsamic vinegar and a splash of coconut oil (it can handle high heat). Sprinkle with Celtic Sea Salt, cover and bake at 400 degrees for one hour. Cool; sprinkle with olive or flax oil and enjoy.

SPICES

If it must be so, then do this: Take...a
little balm and a little honey,
spices.... —GENESIS 43:11

Spices are mentioned several times throughout the Bible, starting from the beginning. Natural God-given herbs and spices add zest to food. Human-made enhancers, though, can confuse the nervous system. Monosodium glutamate (MSG) is probably the most notorious of all. If you are sensitive to MSG, common in Chinese food, it can be a sign of a vitamin B6 deficiency.

Day 113

DR. BOB'S COOKING SECRET

And make me savory food, such as I love, and bring it to me that I may eat, that my soul may bless you before I die. —GENESIS 27:4

A secret weapon used to create a luscious meal is love. Cook with an emotional mindset of love. My friend, a certified nutritional consultant and cookbook author says, "The love permeates through the food." Add love to all the meals you prepare. Organic vanilla extract can be added to any food—be creative. Plan a special meal with love.

WE USE GARLIC

We remember...the garlic. —NUMBERS 11:5

Garlic had medicinal properties that were not found in the "odorless" plants. It is often referred to as Chinese or even Russian penicillin. Garlic has been found to stimulate natural protection against tumor cells. It also provides the liver with a certain amount of protection against chemicals that cause cancer. Even though garlic attacks tumor cells, it is harmless to normal, healthy body cells. Although bad breath from fresh garlic can be a little repelling, it can lower blood pressure, lower cholesterol, and cleanse the blood of impurities.

ROASTED GARLIC

I like to roast garlic in a clay roaster. Then I squeeze the garlic flesh from the clove and spread it on bread with olive or flax oil. Roast cloves of garlic in a covered dish in one fourth inch of water for one hour at 400 degrees. Spread on bread or add to salads and side dishes. Store in an airtight container.

Day 116

DR. BOB'S GRILL TIPS

Then they shall eat the flesh on that night; roasted in fire, with unleavened bread and with bitter herbs they shall eat it. —EXODUS 12:8

I enjoy grilling. I normally grill chicken at a medium setting using a gas grill and add poultry seasoning along with Celtic Sea Salt. Season fresh meat with Celtic Sea Salt, poultry seasoning, or Italian dressing. The cooked items will keep for a few days, stored in airtight containers.

BASTING ON THE GRILL

You can make your own barbecue sauce with sugar-free catsup, chili sauce, and maple syrup or honey. Brush it on with a paint brush while cooking over low heat. Tenderloin meats (beef, lamb, or turkey) are juicy when first grilled at an extremely high temperature to create an outer crust, keeping the juice inside, then lowering the heat to cook thoroughly. I also grill vegetables; brushing on olive oil after they have warmed 10 or 15 minutes. Grilled onions with olive oil are a nice extra side dish.

SEE MORE, EAT MORE

The larger the serving size, the more you're likely to eat. If you're trying to cut calories, shrink your servings. Some suggestions: order a small portion, split a dish with someone, or stash half of what you're served in a doggie bag before you start eating.

DESIGNING DINNER

I would suggest you journal what you eat for at least one month if you contend with sinus issues, skin challenges, pain syndromes, and bowel dysfunction; these systems are impacted by food and the environment. The saying "one person's passion is another person's poison" has to do with what you are putting in and on your body. In the ever-changing world of toxic chemicals used as herbicides and pesticides compounded with the unwise acceptance of genetically-engineered or modified food, you would do your best to keep up with the latest research from independent sources (that is, information not presented by the food manufactures).

Dr. Robert DeMaria

"WHAT CAN I EAT?"

*And out of the ground the Lord God made
every tree grow that is pleasant to the sight
and good for food....* —GENESIS 2:9

You can eat anything you want—as long as it rots. We live in a toxic environment. People, in their ignorance, have created food items that have a long shelf life, increasing profits but decreasing healthiness. Eat food that you prepare from living, whole food ingredients, preferably organic. God made food without chemicals to fuel the system. Human-made food causes the machine (you) to misfire and get sick!

Day 121

BUTTERNUT SQUASH

Butternut squash is one of the easiest and tastiest dishes to make. Set your oven at 350 degrees. Spray olive oil on the bottom of a glass baking dish. Cut the butternut squash in half. Add a touch of water and cover. Bake 45 minutes or until tender. Serve hot with olive oil. Very good!

Day 122

"WHERE'S THE BEEF?"

*And you shall do to Ai and its king as
you did to Jericho and its king. Only
its spoil and its **cattle** you shall take as
booty for yourselves....* —JOSHUA 8:2

Beef is healthy, especially if you focus
on the flesh and not the cover fat. Beef
was not one of the forbidden foods in the
Bible. Attempt to obtain beef from a natural, organic source. Chemical-free, grass-fed
beef is a good source of Omega 3 fats. Pork
is not to be classified with beef.

Day 123

SMART EATING

You need to be aware of the tenderizers and sources of flavor additives used to flavor your favorite dishes. I have found by trial and error that when I have eaten beef at a restaurant and wake up hot, sweaty, or thirsty, I know my body is working overtime to process the chemical tenderizer assault. I generally avoid eating beef when I am out for dinner.

Day 124

COMBATING INFLAMMATION

What you eat, drink, and smoke causes inflammation. Sugar, dairy, too much red meat, trans fat, and soda create an inflammatory state in your blood vessels. Focus on flax oil and olive oil, brown rice syrup in baked goods, almond, rice, or coconut milk, chicken, turkey, fish, and herbal tea or water. Eat fresh vegetables daily. Avoid overeating inflammation-producing sugar and dairy products.

CHOOSE NATURAL MEAT

I encourage consumption of meat products from a natural, pure source. How an animal is handled affects the taste. You want the animal raised so its natural immunity is enhanced. Does the beef, chicken, turkey, or lamb you eat cause digestive distress? It may be the chemicals given to the animals. Do some research; there are excellent sources of safe animal tissue. Evaluate your digestive response to any animal tissue you consume. Vary sources if you experience distress. Be mindful of marinated products.

SAFE FISH?

Fish is an excellent source of protein and fat essential for optimum brain function. Avoid unclean fish like swordfish, shark, lumpfish, and European flat fish, because they have the highest levels of mercury and pesticides. Instead, choose deep-water ocean fish, as they are an excellent source of Omega 3 fat.

SEAFOOD AND STROKE

E at seafood at least once or twice a week if possible. (You may only need one serving a month to reduce your risk of stroke, but earlier studies suggested that eating one or two servings a week can reduce your risk of heart disease.) If you don't eat fish, try to add flax oil to boost your intake of alpha-linolenic acid, which your body may convert to the Omega 3 fats that are in fish oil.

WHO IS GUIDING YOUR SHIP?

*...no longer be children **tossed to and fro** and carried about with every wind of doctrine, by the trickery of men....* —EPHESIANS 4:14

In the beginning of God's Word, we are advised to eat living food with seed. My advice to you is to eat whole food such as broccoli, cabbage, green and yellow beans, squash, celery—real food. Jesus also ate lamb, figs, fish, and bread. I suggest that, even in your hectic life, you plan your meals ahead of time, focusing on the use of organic items. No plan is a plan to fail. Plan and purchase products to create one week of meals.

A LIVING SACRIFICE

God wants us to present our bodies a living sacrifice, holy, acceptable to God "which is your reasonable service. And do not be conformed to this world, but be transformed by the renewing of your mind" (Rom. 12:1-2). This is a mandate to keep your body in good, working order. Allow God to be the guide of your ship. Look to His Word for direction.

A NEW BURGER

Don't be tricked into believing that processed food is wholesome. Try something new, for example: ground turkey thigh and breast mixed with an organic egg, sugar-free catsup, bread crumbs, and Italian herbs. Press into a baking dish and cover. Bake at 350 degrees for one hour or until tender and brown. Slice and freeze. Take slices out on days when you are pressed for time. This is a delicious fast-food substitute when combined with your favorite sauce, in salads, or eaten alone.

WHAT CAME WITH DINNER?

Americans do not like to accept the fact that we have parasites living inside our bodies. But it has been estimated that there are more parasitic infections acquired in this country (the United States) than in Africa. When a person is afflicted with parasites, the body's supply of nutrients is depleted to the point that supplementation of all nutrients is necessary to restore normal health. We use a natural enzyme and sulfur product to control parasite growth. Parasites do not like sulfur sourced naturally from eggs, onion, garlic, and cruciferous veggies. Completely cook all food. Do not eat raw meat or fish.

Day 132

ONE FOOD AT A TIME

When you go out to dinner with an influential person, mind your manners: Don't gobble your food, don't talk with your mouth full. And don't stuff yourself; bridle your appetite. —PROVERBS 23:2 THE MESSAGE

Do you suffer with digestive distress? Do you have a relentless, gnawing pain in the pit of your stomach that creates fear and anxiety and interferes with life? A leading, missed cause of digestive pain is eating different food in layers that the body is not capable of processing. One such example is starch. Starchy veggies and grains are best eaten alone, not with animal protein. Protein needs an acid environment; potatoes are best digested with alkaline. Eat starches and greens alone, not in combination with other foods.

EAT IN PEACE

Better is a dinner of herbs where love is, than a fatted calf with hatred. —PROVERBS 15:17

God's Word encourages you to eat your morsels of food in peace without distress. Chew your food long and slowly. This will reduce the amount of work your stomach and pancreas need to do. Emotional distress can impair the release of these natural digestive aides resulting in malabsorption. Do not eat while you are on the run in your car. Always take time to break bread around the table—even if it is only one healthy, fast food meal a day.

STIR-FRY

*So Gideon went in and prepared a young
goat, and unleavened bread from an ephah
of flour. The meat he put in a basket, and
he put the broth in a pot....* —JUDGES 6:19

Stir-fry meals are simple, easy, and
healthy, depending on what you choose
to prepare. Purchase a wok that is electric
or one that can be warmed on top of the
stove. Purchase organic vegetable broth as a
base. There is a wheat-free soy sauce called
Organic Tamari made by San-J. I also add
sesame seeds, Celtic Sea Salt, and fresh
herbs such as basil, chives, and parsley. Simmer over medium heat, cooking until tender.
Simultaneously prepare flat rice noodles.

CLEAN OUT YOUR FRIDGE!

Plan a stir-fry meal—a handy way to clean out your refrigerator. This is a healthy alternative to any fast food. Consider avoiding nightshade veggies and gluten-based flours in all meal planning, including stir-frying, if you continue to chronically experience pain, skin problems, headache, fatigue, fibromyalgia, or digestive symptoms.

BODY FERTILIZER

*A certain man had a fig tree planted
in his vineyard, and he came seeking
fruit on it and found none. ..."Sir, let it
alone this year also, until I dig around
it and fertilize it." —LUKE 13:6,8*

Not feeling at peak performance? Journal food patterns for one week. Wheat, corn, dairy, sugar, nightshades, alcohol, and citrus are common energy zappers. Look at the labels of all fruits and vegetables. A PLU number on the label starting with 9 indicates organic, and an 8 indicates genetically-engineered. All other numbers are considered conventional, which means they have herbicides and pesticides.

MEDITERRANEAN MIX

In a study of more than 22,000 adults in Greece, those who ate a more traditional Mediterranean diet had a lower death rate (largely due to fewer deaths from heart disease and cancer) than others. There's plenty of evidence from other studies to recommend less fatty meat and dairy and more vegetables, fruits, beans, fish, and unsaturated oils like olive and canola.

Day 138

DRUGLESS CARE

...The head—CHRIST—FROM WHOM THE
WHOLE BODY, JOINED *and knit together by
what every joint supplies, according to the
effective working by which every part does
its share, causes growth of the body for the
edifying of itself in love.* —Ephesians 4:15-16

How would you like to get healthy and
stay healthy without medication? Sound
farfetched? It's not. An ounce of prevention
is worth a pound of cure. Common conditions requiring medical assistance including
antibiotics or pain relievers can be traced
to what is being eaten and, over time, toxic
accumulation. Choose items with complex-
based sweeteners like brown rice syrup or
the herb stevia.

Day 139

BEANS

[They] *brought beds and basins, earthen vessels and wheat, barley and flour, parched grain and beans...* —SECOND SAMUEL 17:28

We have been blessed with a wide variety of foods. Diversification is a wise approach. Avoid eating the same choices all the time. Eat string green or yellow beans. They are a source of vitamins, minerals, iron, Omega 3 fat, and protein.

Day 140

MORE BEANS

Organic black beans in a can are a great source of fiber and vegetable protein, which can easily be added to a mixed green salad. Lima beans mixed with yellow corn and onions along with a dash of Paul Newman's Oil and Vinegar dressing creates a colorful side dish. Create a new mindset of options. Add some beans to your salad or as a side dish!

HEALTHY DIGESTION

Do you not yet understand that whatever enters the mouth goes into the stomach and is eliminated? —MATTHEW 15:17

Continued consumption of toxic food substances eventually will lead to a state of poor health. The body will absorb nutrients from whatever you consume. Do not be fooled. Continued inappropriate choices will result in auto-intoxification, which actually means you've put yourself in a state of toxicity. Some common body signals include sinusitis, ear wax, diarrhea, colitis, skin rashes, acne, arthritis, asthma, psoriasis, pain, kidney failure, liver disease, and eye disease.

Day 142

OUR TOXIC WORLD

Many, if not most, modern health conditions are a result of toxicity. Here is the million-dollar question: Do you take an antihistamine or pain pill to mask the symptoms of poor choices, or do you make life-enhancing decisions? Pharmaceuticals do not cure. They modify symptoms. What a smoke screen! Avoid toxic, processed food.

Don't Be Foolish!

*But the natural man does not receive
the things of the Spirit of God, for
they are foolishness to him; nor can he
know them, because they are spiritually
discerned.* —First Corinthians 2:14

Do not eat food that does not rot. Margarine is not a food, and aspirin is not a vitamin. Soda is loaded with chemicals, especially phosphoric acid, that can lead to osteoporosis and cavities. Artificial "heart-healthy Egg Beaters" confuse the system. Processed cheese does not mold in the sun. White enriched bread will never be as good as whole wheat. Cow's milk is for cows; human milk is for humans.

DR. BOB'S SUPPER

There they made Him a supper; and Martha served, but Lazarus was one of those who sat at the table with Him. —JOHN 12:2

Planning is the key component for eating at home. Generally, I focus on vegetables and protein. I grill on a gas burner or a George Foreman Grill. I brush chicken, turkey, or duck with Paul Newman's Oil and Vinegar Dressing and grill them in lettuce so the meat stays moist. Asparagus is awesome on the grill, brushed with olive oil. We also cut up and cook onions with olive oil on the grill. Protein is similar to adding a log to the fire. Stoke your fire with nuts and lean meat and fish.

THE DAIRY DIET MYTH

"Drink milk...lose weight" say the ads. Low-fat (or nonfat) milk, yogurt, and cheese can help lower blood pressure and boost calcium intake. But don't expect them to keep you slim.

DINNER

Your goal is to eat a light, late afternoon or evening meal focusing on the mid-level glycemic range. Focus on fish, animal, or plant protein. Eat steamed, raw, or lightly sautéed vegetables. Consume animal proteins separately from grains or starches. Eat at home with friends or family rather than frequenting restaurants or fast food joints.

Identifying
Troublesome Foods

I have successfully helped patients with chronic conditions by suggesting they have a food sensitivity or IgG4 blood spot test. I have discovered most patients and worldwide clients literally have digestive distress in their intestines permitting undigested food particles to be transported in the blood and lymph systems. The protein particles from the undigested foods create an alarm, and the patient suffers with histamine reactions including stuffy runny noses, headache, lung congestion, loose stools, and pain syndromes, even memory issues and fatigue. You are what you eat and digest.

SWEETS AND DESSERTS

There are times when you will crave or want something sweet. Chromium supplementation reduces the sugar desire. Protein helps keep blood sugar levels steady without fluctuations. Organic raisins are an alternative to candy. Avoid a consistent diet of sweet fruit and snacks. They can cause pain by stressing the organ that makes natural cortisone, the adrenal gland.

GLYCEMIC INDEX

In practical terms, the glycemic index means that each food has the ability to raise blood glucose to variable degrees. The greater the blood glucose, the greater the insulin response. Thus, we want to choose food with low glycemic indices. Foods with low glycemic indices may enhance satiety, and foods with low glycemic indices may increase athletic performance.

THE RIGHT BALANCE

Your body can't produce enough digestive enzymes without the right balance of minerals and B vitamins. Compensating for your sweet tooth with extra healthy foods may be a losing battle since your body is no longer digesting or assimilating food efficiently. Eating sugar puts stress on digestion. Poor digestion can lead to allergies. Sugar consumption results in poor health.

SWEETENERS TO AVOID

What about other refined sugars? Brown sugar is simply refined sugar that is sprayed with molasses to make it appear more whole. Turbinado sugar gives the illusion of health, but is just one step away from white sugar. Turbinado is made from 95 percent sucrose (table sugar). It skips only the final filtration stage of sugar refining with little difference in nutritional value. I would say no to sucralose (Splenda™) and Agave products.

Corn Syrup

Corn syrup is found everywhere. It is used in everything from bouillon cubes to spaghetti sauce and even in some "natural" juices. Corn syrup processed from cornstarch is almost as sweet as refined sugar and is absorbed quickly by your blood. Corn-derived sweeteners pose other problems: they often contain high levels of pesticide residues that are genetically modified and are common allergy producers. This is a cheap and plentiful sweetener often used in soft drinks, candy, and baked goods.

Day 153

ASPARTAME

Aspartame, which is a common synthetic sweetener, affects the nervous system and brain in a very negative way. Aspartame is made from two proteins, or amino acids, which give it super-sweetness. Aspartame has many harmful effects: behavior changes in children, headaches, dizziness, epileptic-like seizures, and bulging of the eyes to name a few. Aspartame is an "excitotoxin," a substance that over-stimulates neurons and causes them to die suddenly (as though they were excited to death). One of the last steps of aspartame metabolism is formaldehyde. The next time you consume diet soda, think. You are literally embalming yourself.

SWEETENERS—THE BEST OF THE NATURALS

Become sugar-savvy! The term natural, as applied to sweeteners, can mean many things. The following recommended sweeteners will provide you with steady energy because they take a long time to digest. Natural choices offer rich flavors, vitamins, and minerals without the ups and downs of refined sugars. Try brown rice syrup, Devansoy™, barley malt syrup, amasake, or stevia.

SUGAR SUBSTITUTES

Sugar substitutes were actually the natural sweeteners of days past, especially honey and maple syrup. Stay away from human-made artificial sweeteners including aspartame and any of the "sugar alcohols" (names ending in "ol"). In health food stores, be alert for sugars disguised as "evaporated cane juice" or "cane juice crystals." These can still cause problems, regardless of what the health food store manager tells you. My patients have seen huge improvements by changing their sugar choices.

Brown Rice Syrup

Your bloodstream absorbs this balanced syrup, high in maltose and complex carbohydrates, slowly and steadily. Brown rice syrup is a natural sweetener for baked goods and hot drinks; it adds subtle sweetness and a rich, butterscotch-like flavor. To get sweetness from starchy brown rice, the magic ingredients are enzymes, but the actual process varies depending on the syrup manufacturer. For a healthy treat, drizzle gently heated rice syrup over popcorn to make natural caramel corn! Store in a cool, dry place.

DEVANSOY

Devansoy is the brand name for powdered brown rice sweetener, which contains the same complex carbohydrates as brown rice syrup as well as a natural plant flavoring.

Barley malt syrup—this sweetener is made much like rice syrup, but it uses sprouted barley to turn grain starches into a complex sweetener that is digested slowly. Use barley malt syrup to add molasses-like flavor and light sweetness to beans, cookies, muffins, and cakes. Store in a cool, dry place.

Day 158

AMASAKE

Amasake is an ancient, Oriental whole-grain sweetener made from cultured brown rice. It has a thick, pudding-like consistency. Baked goods benefit from amasake's subtle sweetness, moisture, and leavening power.

STEVIA

Stevia is a sweet South American herb that has been safely used by many cultures for centuries. Extensive scientific studies confirm these ancient claims to safety. However, the FDA has approved it only when labeled as a dietary supplement, not as a sweetener. Advocates consider stevia to be one of the healthiest sweeteners as well as a tonic for healing skin. Stevia is 150 to 400 times sweeter than white sugar, has no calories, and can actually regulate blood sugar levels. Unrefined stevia has a molasses-like flavor; refined stevia (popular in Japan) has less flavor and nutrients.

FRUITSOURCE®

This brand-name sweetener combines the sweetness of grape juice concentrate with the complex carbohydrates of brown rice syrup. FruitSource is light amber in color and 80 percent as sweet as white sugar. Look for FruitSource in liquid and granulated form. Liquid Plus, a similar product, better matches the sweetness of white sugar. Whichever form you choose, the options are better for your blood sugar than refined sugar!

WHOLE FRUIT

For baking, try fruit purees, dried fruit, and cooked fruit sauces or butters. The less water remaining in a fruit, the more concentrated its flavor and sugar content. You'll find fiber and naturally balanced nutrients in whole fruits like apples, bananas, and apricots. To add mild sweetness and moisture to baked goods, mix in the magic of mashed winter squashes, sweet potatoes, and carrots!

Day 162

HONEY

Honey is mostly made of glucose and fructose and is up to twice as sweet as white sugar. Honey enters the bloodstream rapidly. Buy raw honey, which still contains some vitamins, minerals, enzymes, and pollen. Honeys vary in color (according to their flower source) and range in strength from mild clover to strong orange blossom. A benefit of eating honey produced in your geographical region is that it may reduce hay fever and allergy symptoms by bolstering your natural immunity.

Maple Syrup

It takes about ten gallons of maple sap to produce one gallon of maple syrup. Like honey, a little goes a long way. Maple syrup is roughly 65 percent sucrose and contains small amounts of trace minerals. Maple syrup has a rich taste and is absorbed fairly quickly into the bloodstream. Select real maple syrup that has no added corn syrup. Also, look for syrups that come from organic producers who don't use formaldehyde to prolong sap flow. Grade A syrups come from the first tapping; they range in color from light to dark amber. Grade B syrups come from the last tapping; they have more minerals and a stronger flavor and color.

Day 164

DATE SUGAR

This sweetener is made from dried, ground dates, is light brown, and has a sugary texture. Date sugar retains many naturally occurring vitamins and minerals, is 65 percent sucrose, and has a fairly rapid affect on blood sugar. Use it in baking in place of brown sugar, but reduce your baking time or temperature in order to prevent premature browning. Store in a cool, dry place.

CONCENTRATED FRUIT JUICE

All concentrates are not created equally. Highly refined juice sweeteners are labeled "modified." These sweeteners, similar to white sugar, have lost both their fruit flavor and their nutrients. Better choices are fruit concentrates that have been evaporated in a vacuum. These retain rich fruit flavors and aromas along with many vitamins and minerals. Carefully read labels on cereal, cookie, jelly, and beverage containers, then choose products with the highest percentage of real fruit juice. Beware of white grape juice concentrates that aren't organic; their pesticide residues can be high!

Day 166

BLACKSTRAP MOLASSES

Molasses, a by-product of sugar production, is a highly-processed simple sugar that enters the bloodstream rapidly. Molasses may also contain chemical residues associated with the growing and refining of white sugar. If you grew up on conventional molasses, your taste buds may have to adjust to the softer bite of blackstrap molasses, which contains high amounts of balancing minerals such as calcium, iron, potassium, magnesium, zinc, copper, and chromium. Use it as a sweetener in cakes, pies, and cookies. Barbados molasses is sweeter and more syrupy than blackstrap; it is perfect for baking, but lacks blackstrap's minerals. (Note: Diabetics should not use any type of molasses.)

BLOOD SUGAR FLUCTUATIONS

Patients who have an issue with blood sugar fluctuations, commonly called hypoglycemia, appear to be more sensitive to sweet fruits. Are you one of those unsuspecting individuals? Here's a question for you. Do you crave bananas, raisins, dried fruit, dates, figs, or grapes? Eliminate them from your diet and focus on greens and protein. For one month, slowly incorporate pears, plums, and one half of an apple back into your diet. Focus on eating veggies for a sweet fruit replacement.

Day 168

CAROB

Carob is a possible replacement for people with chocolate allergies. Carob does have a fair amount of protein as well as some calcium and phosphorous, and it does have B vitamins and minerals. Carob is available in tablet, powder, syrup, and wafer forms. Make sure you read labels and look at the source of sweeteners in the products with carob. Don't be fooled. Evaporated cane juice or crystals is still sugar. Carob serves as an excellent illustration that excessive use of any "natural" substance can have its own health risks. Carob chips are an option for milk chocolate. Read labels, avoid sugar.

HONEY

Patients do not appear to get addicted to honey like they do refined sugar. However, honey does cause left neck pain. The pancreas must do some type of extra work to process it. Natural honey from a local beekeeper promotes health. Honey has over 150 ingredients, such as collagen with a protein called proline. My suggestion is to slowly divert your sugar cravings to honey. Plan to take a drive in your area to find and secure a local source of honey from a beekeeper. Ask for a source at your local health food store.

Day 170

SPIRITUAL ARM WRESTLING

*All things are lawful for me, but all things
are not helpful. All things are lawful for me,
but I will not be brought under the power
of any.* —FIRST CORINTHIANS 6:12

Our bodies are the temple of the Holy
Spirit who, if we have asked Jesus into
our hearts, is living in us. We are not our
own, for we were bought at a price. Therefore, we must glorify God in our bodies and
in our spirits. Sugar paralyzes the immune
system, thus promoting death. Satan came
to steal, kill, and destroy, and I believe sugar
has the potential to sabotage our walk with
the Lord. Add whole food chromium to
your supplement routine if you crave sugar.

MORE MAPLE SYRUP

Imagine the delight on the taste buds of the first person who sampled the initial batch of boiled sap. Maple syrup from the tree (without high fructose corn syrup added to it, as in commercial products) is a viable alternative to refined, white crystalline sugar. Like honey, a little goes a long way. Select real maple syrup that has no added high fructose corn syrup. Use maple syrup as an alternative to sugar. One fourth cup of maple syrup is equivalent to one half cup of sugar.

LIMIT YOUR
FRUIT SUGAR

Your body requires a limited amount of all of the primary building blocks: carbohydrates, fats, and proteins. When you focus on and consume the sweeter fruits or carbs, your body will convert them to fat. Limit sweet fruits like bananas, raisins, and grapes. Avoid or limit all dried fruit, including apricots, prunes, dates, and figs.

Managing Cortisol

Refined food depletes cortisol, a hormone from the adrenals, which is required to shut off insulin when protein in the diet is low. When insulin stays elevated, your extra carbs are converted to fat around the belly in males and buttocks in females. Over time, with a breakdown of adrenal and pancreas function, exhaustion occurs. Once exhausted, the body no longer burns carbs effectively and, therefore, cannot provide fuel for the body.

THE DANGER OF SUGAR ALTERNATIVES

Every few years a newer, safer, human-made sugar alternative promises to be sweet and safe. Nothing made by people will ever be safe enough for people to consume. All the commercial brands eventually create a negative toxic situation including damage to the liver, which processes and filters all chemicals. Increase chromium supplement intake if you crave sweets. Switch to grape juice spritzers as an alternative to sugary corn syrup soda.

RED ALERT

High fructose corn syrup (HFCS) is detrimental to your health. HFCS can deplete leptin, which is a hormone used by the body to signal you are full. Eating foods with HFCS, even applesauce or a beverage, may be the reason you are always hungry. Leptin levels can be assessed using noninvasive galvanic skin response biocommunication technology. Do not be fooled by the word fructose—it's safe in whole foods, but alone as HFCS it can lead to obesity. Read food product labels.

SIDE PAIN

And the Lord God caused a deep sleep to fall on Adam, and he slept; and He took one of his ribs, and closed up the flesh in its place. Then the rib which the Lord God had taken from man He made into a woman.... —GENESIS 2:21-22

Did you ever have severe, intense pain that is worse when breathing, often on the left side, the kind of pain that imitates a heart attack? What you eat, especially sweet foods and drinks, can weaken supporting structures, possibly resulting in the displacement of a rib, causing relentless pain. Avoid sugar, bananas, raisins, and grapes that could cause rib pain.

WE LOVE SWEETS

L et's be real. We all like sweet foods. The challenge is to not let the sweets have us. Sugar-loaded alcohol enslaves people in a devastating yoke. Ice cream can create an addiction, resulting in unsuspecting symptoms including sinusitis, headaches, pancreas stress, acne, and colon issues. Be mindful of the additives used to flavor ice cream. Some of the artificial flavors are potent poisons powerful enough to cause liver, kidney, pancreas, and heart damage. Whole cream without additives or chemical enhancers is the logical choice. Read ingredient labels.

THE DANGER OF DOUGHNUTS

Let's have a little doughnut talk. The average doughnut adds a minimum of 300 calories. The trans fat alone will do enough damage to your cell membranes and nervous system to cripple your body's ability to communicate for up to 102 days (the double half-life of trans fat). Replace breakfast Do-Nots with quinoa, a gluten-free oatmeal replacement, or short grain brown rice with almonds, applesauce, and cinnamon.

STEVIA—SWEETENER

...Take and eat it; and it; [synthetic sweeteners] *will make your stomach bitter, but it will be as sweet as honey in your mouth.* —REVELATION 10:9

Sugar is a secret killer in America. Sugar is lurking in packaged entrees, condiments, sauces, dressings, and soups. It can be found in nearly every imaginable commercially available item in conventional grocery stores. Tip: Always make a shopping list and never shop when you are hungry. Read labels as though you were on a reconnaissance mission—like a trained soldier. Eat as a cave man would—whole food, grains, veggies, and fruit.

THE SWEETEST OPTION

Not recognized as a sweetener by the U.S. government, stevia, a South American herb, is 200 to 300 times sweeter than regular sugar. Stevia has no calories, is suitable for diabetics, does not cause cavities, and is heat stable, which means it can be used for cooking and baking. Stevia is a great alternative to synthetic sweeteners. It blends easily with honey, and it has been safely consumed in many countries around the world for decades.

GROWING OUR SWEETS

Stevia grows about 18 inches tall with small, narrow leaves. I pluck stevia leaves from the top down and dry them in a piloted oven or dehydrator, then store the dried leaves in an airtight container. The leaves are then easily powdered in a blender. Sprinkle the green herb on any item you generally sweeten with sugar or substitute. Splenda is chlorinated sucrose derivatives. It enlarges the liver and kidneys and shrinks the thymus. Plant some stevia in your garden!

SUPPOSEDLY HEALTHY FOODS

Sport drinks and power bars commonly found in athletic facilities, conventional grocery stores, and health food stores are stealthy candy bars. Be aware of "evaporated organic cane juice crystals," which is sugar in disguise. I avoid all human-made synthetic sugars. Manitol, sorbitol, and xylitol are alcohol-based sweeteners marketed as "sugar free," which create additional stress to the detox system. Seek grape juice sweetener, brown rice syrup, stevia, honey or pear sweetener as natural sourced sweeteners. Read labels; do not be fooled by organic evaporated cane crystals.

Day 183

PASS THE HONEY

Have you found honey? Eat only as much as you need, lest you be filled with it and vomit. —PROVERBS 25:16

Honey is talked about throughout the Bible. Honey can be an excellent source of a natural sweetener, but I have seen major issues with overdoing honey similar to what I see with sugar consumption. Honey is 95 percent sucrose, and sucrose is sugar. No, honey is not white table sugar, but I have treated patients with chronic pain who use honey as a sugar substitute and suffer with sugar headaches, pain syndromes, mood swings, depression, and so forth just like those who consume sugar.

CONSUME HONEY

Eat honey from your geographic region, but go easy on it. Do not use it every day. In fact, try going without sweets for a few weeks. You will feel better! Only consume non-processed honey that is gathered by honey bees from your region.

A HEALTHY IMMUNE SYSTEM

Your immune system is working 24/7. A properly functioning digestive system is critical for immune function. In the liver, a group of cells called kupffer cells neutralize unwanted bacteria, viruses, parasites, and even cancer cells. Sugar, when you eat it, paralyzes the immune system for hours. One white blood cell (WBC) can handle fourteen bacteria in half an hour. Consuming a soda handcuffs the WBC so it can only handle ten, and eating a brownie reduces WBC activity to five. Enjoying Grandma's apple pie or a banana split sabotages the WBC to handle only one bacterium. My suggestion is to polish your armor with healthy food. Sugar tarnishes your protective covering.

Day 186

LABEL READERS

...When it is evening you say, "It will be fair weather, for the sky is red"; and in the morning, "It will be foul weather today, for the sky is red..." —MATTHEW 16:2-3

Buyer beware! When you go into a health food store or health food department in a large conventional chain, read the ingredients on the label. Evaporated, organic cane juice is still sugar. Raw, organic cane crystals are sugar. Do not be duped. Write a letter or voice your opinion to these companies or the store that has them on their shelves. Read the label on your "healthy" power bar. It may contain hidden sugar sources.

KNOWLEDGE IS POWER

My people are destroyed for lack of knowledge.... —HOSEA 4:6

Sugar handcuffs your white blood cells from performing their job. A can of soda with nine-and-a-half teaspoons of sugar can depress your immune system by up to 25 percent for five to six hours. And that is just one can! People who eat sugar are always sick and never 100 percent healthy. Stevia, honey, or maple syrup are alternative sweeteners to sugar.

THE DOWNSIDE TO SNACKING

Continuous "grazing" may keep your blood sugar steady, but also stresses the digestive system. Focus on snacks that do not cause a large insulin release. The Glycemic Index midrange is best. Sweets can be addictive, resulting in extra pounds and an underlying cause of pain.

Day 189

DIGESTION—NOT INDIGESTION

Jesus talked about digestion in His parables. You are not only what you eat, but also what you digest and absorb. Poor digestion can result in food that is not broken down to proper size. Food enters and leaves the body. What you decide to eat becomes you. It is serious. Regular daily elimination is essential for optimal well-being. You would do best to eat fresh, organic fiber foods to assist colon elimination.

Day 190

YOUR LIVER—
YOUR LIFELINE

Till an arrow struck his liver....
—PROVERBS 7:23

The liver is an incredible organ with hundreds of known functions. It is so highly regarded in Eastern and Asian cultures that newlyweds figuratively exchange livers instead of the heart as we are accustomed to in Western societies. Add Dr. Bob's ABCs to your daily routine, one half of an Apple, a portion of grated raw or baked Beets, and a moderate Carrot for optimal liver function.

YOUR BODY'S FILTER

The liver is commonly seen as the literal "oil filter" of the body—but it does so much more. Reserves of blood are stored in the liver along with fat soluble vitamins, including A, D, E, and K. Your liver creates bile necessary for proper metabolism of fat. Kupffer cells are active in a healthy liver, seeking and destroying unhealthy invaders, including cancer cells and parasites. Toxins (modern-day arrows) from the air, water, and processed foods and drinks stress the liver.

"And Make Bread for Yourself"

Also take for yourself wheat, barley, beans, lentils, millet, and spelt; put them into one vessel, and make bread of them for yourself.... —Ezekiel 4:9

Craving bread can be a body signal that you may have a wheat and/or yeast sensitivity. Vary the grains in the bread you use. Try spelt, millet, rice, oat, or barley flour bread. Rotate your bread choices to include a sprouted grain variety.

DANIEL'S MENU

But Daniel purposed in his heart that he would not defile himself [eat pork] *with the portion of the king's delicacies, nor with the wine which he drank....* —DANIEL 1:8

Daniel was a very wise young man. He had God's favor on his life and the wisdom not to choose items consumed by the kings and royalty. Food consumed in Daniel's day was not refrigerated. Fruit, vegetables, and grains are generally easily digested and do not create an unhealthy digestive environment. I wonder if Daniel had blood type A. I have noticed that patients with blood type A have distress with meat products.

Day 194

"Mmmmm Good"

Oh, taste and see that the Lord is good.... —Psalm 34:8

My clinical experience suggests that another common cause of not being able to taste is a zinc deficiency. Zinc can be depleted by stress or eating certain grains and protein sources such as wheat and soy. When you have a zinc deficiency, you may notice white spots on your nails, large pores on your face, and excessive scarring at the site of an injury. Memory lapses? Avoid zinc-depleting wheat and soy. Snack on fresh, raw pumpkin seeds.

Day 195

"OH, I ATE THE WHOLE THING!"

Have you found honey? Eat only as much as you need, lest you be filled with it and vomit. —PROVERBS 25:16

Digestive distress is one of the leading reasons why people take medications. I encourage my patients not to drink water or fluids with meals. Fluids dilute or weaken the digestive process and most people do not have enough stomach acid. The diminished acid state, with the presence of fluids, results in poor digestion. You literally can have a compost pile in your stomach, which creates an inorganic acid that people dissolve with antacids, which only compound the problem.

HEALTHY FOOD COMBINATIONS

Be aware how you combine foods. I recommend protein with non-starch items. Proteins with greens are a good choice. Protein needs an acid environment. Starches need an alkaline (such as baking soda) environment. I also instruct my patients to eat fruit alone and not to end a meal with it. Eaten with food, the fruit decomposes for hours literally breaking down into alcohol and stressing your system. Do not drink sparkling or "still" water or clear broths with your meals—it dilutes the digestive acid. Drink water before and after, not during the meal.

VEGGIES AND DIABETES

Yellow-orange and green leafy vegetables may lower the risk of diabetes in overweight women. Eat nutrient-packed yellow-orange vegetables like carrots, sweet potatoes, and yellow squash and green leafy vegetables like spinach, kale, and lettuce.

DIGESTION STARTS IN THE MOUTH

...honey and milk are under your tongue.... —SONG OF SOLOMON 4:11

Chew your food long and slowly. The more you chew your food, the better the digestion. Starch digestion requires enzymes that are released by saliva glands in the chewing process. Nutrients are quickly absorbed in the mouth. You might even want to chew your whole food vitamins with the exception of ascorbic acid.

HEALTHY TEETH

Do you have silver-color, mercury-based amalgam fillings in your mouth? Mercury is very toxic and interferes with the production of digestive juices released from the parotid glands located in your throat. I encourage my patients to take chlorophyll capsules and parotid tissue (an animal-based extract) if they have a mouth full of fillings and have allergies. It would be best to have your amalgams removed by a skilled, experienced dentist.

WHAT IS THE GLYCEMIC INDEX?

And they gave him a piece of a cake of figs and two clusters of raisins. So when he had eaten, his strength came back to him; for he had eaten no bread nor drunk water for three days and three nights. —FIRST SAMUEL 30:12

When David fed on the Egyptian slave's figs and raisins, he was revived. In the New Testament, Saul, prior to being Paul, did not eat for several days before he was filled with the Holy Spirit. The physical person requires fuel just as the spirit person needs to be filled with the Holy Spirit. Acts 9:19 says, "So when [Saul] had received food, he was strengthened…."

FUELING OUR SYSTEM

Our bodies require fuel to flourish. How fast the fuel enters the system can promote or deplete life. You can be on a roller coaster of health with peaks and valleys with headaches, depression, anxiety, pain, dizziness, digestive distress, and more depending on the carbohydrates you choose to eat. A low GI diet results in a smaller rise in blood glucose after meals, which promotes weight loss, helps you stay full longer, and prolongs physical endurance. The fuel you put in your machine affects physical performance. Reduce the amount of white potatoes you eat, especially if you notice the correlation of mid-back pain after eating them. Yams and sweet potatoes do not generally create the same insulin rush.

BODY DE-GREASER: BILE

...my bile is poured on the ground....
—LAMENTATIONS 2:11

Optimal liver function is necessary for bile to flow freely. I encourage my patients to eat at least half an apple daily along with organic beets, either grated raw or baked and diced, not canned or pickled. Bile can become thick and concentrated forming gallstones. I encourage patients who have had gallbladder surgery to supplement their diet with a bile salt. Eating fiber, apples, and beets facilitates the removal of bile from the body.

DON'T WORRY—BE HAPPY

Martha, Martha, you are worried and troubled about many things. But one thing is needed, and Mary has chosen that good part, which will not be taken away from her. —LUKE 10:41-42

A very common deficiency in Americans today is complex vitamin B. It's not easy to get real B vitamins in the American diet. First of all, the richest source of these vitamins is brewer's yeast (not exactly a staple of the average American). Other sources of B vitamins are whole grains, lamb, nuts, eggs, beans, and brown rice.

NIGHTSHADES

There is a classification of food items called nightshades, that in and of themselves are not harmful or bad. They have a substance that is part of their makeup called solanine. Solanine is an irritant to the liver. Your liver needs to be functioning optimally in order for you not to have pain or inflammation caused by the nightshades. Commonly consumed nightshades include tomatoes, white potatoes, eggplant, and green pepper. Eating too many tomatoes with a congested liver can result in intense pain for some. Raw, grated, organic beets or mixed greens promote liver health. Substitute yams and sweet potatoes for white potatoes.

OUR BODY'S SHIELD

The immune system is a shield against invaders. Our bodies are under a tight balance or ecosystem. Tipping the scale can create functional stress and may create toxic overload. Your lymphatic system does not have a pump like the vascular network. It depends on muscle movement. The lymph system is your sewage and street cleaning department that carries and destroys unfriendly cells, used cells, and organisms. Halitosis, or bad breath, may be a sign of sluggish digestion and poor lymphatic drainage. Combine your foods wisely; reduce liquids with meals.

Eat Healthy, Stay Healthy

Magnesium may protect against colorectal cancer, according to a study of more than 61,000 Swedish women. Eat more fruits, vegetables, whole grains, and beans—all of which are rich in magnesium. Multivitamins rarely contain a day's worth—320 milligrams for women and 420 milligrams for men—because the amount needed wouldn't fit into a single tablet.

FIBER CLEAN

Jacob gave Esau bread and stew of lentils.... —GENESIS 25:34

Fiber-rich food, like beans and legumes, cleanse the small finger-like projecting villi in the digestive system. Fiber helps lower blood cholesterol and stabilizes blood sugar. Beet and oatmeal fiber prevent colon cancer, constipation, hemorrhoids, obesity, and many other disorders. It is also good for removing certain toxic metals from the body. Because the refining process has removed much of the natural fiber from our foods, the typical American diet is lacking fiber.

HANDLING PRODUCE

When eating organic produce, leave the washed skin on the apples and eggplant. I would suggest, since eggplant is a nightshade, that you do not eat it more than once or twice a month if you have emotional challenges and anger. The liver is the organ of anger and must be functioning optimally to process the nightshade family.

A VEGETABLE GARDEN

For the land which you go to possess is not like the land of Egypt from which you have come, where you sowed your seed and watered it by foot, as a vegetable garden. —DEUTERONOMY 11:10

Gardens are good for you physically and emotionally. I have patients who spend hours in their gardens. It is very therapeutic. Decide what you want to grow; then find an organic source of plants and seeds. Find a sunny location for your garden. Obtain quality soil and add compost throughout the year. Put the residue from juicing in your compost.

Day 210

CASTOR OIL

So he went to him and bandaged his wounds,
pouring on oil and wine; and he set him
on his own animal, brought him to an inn,
and took care of him. —LUKE 10:34

Oil can be a healing agent for many conditions. The properties in God-made organic, natural oil are best (no solvents in the refining process). I generally eat flax and olive oil daily. From my experience helping even the most serious health conditions, I have found the oil processing liver to be a pivotal factor for restoring health. Castor oil itself has natural healing physiology. It contains natural levels of pain-relieving, health-promoting fat tissue hormones called Prostaglandin 3 (PG3).

CASTOR OIL PACK

Weekly castor oil pack application to the liver area promotes function. Put castor oil on a piece of wool—we use unbleached lamb's wool—and warm it in the oven for ten minutes at 300 degrees. Place a heating pad in a plastic bag, and cover the floor or couch with plastic or a towel. Dress in a set of clothes that you don't mind getting oily. Put the warm castor-oiled wool on your lower right rib cage and belly. Put the heating pad (high setting) on top of the wool for one hour. Rest. Apply this castor oil pack once a week for six months. You can do it as often as you like after that. This procedure revitalizes liver function. Remember to drink water and avoid toxic food and beverages.

EVERY PART DOES ITS SHARE

...Christ—FROM WHOM THE WHOLE BODY,
JOINED *and knit together by what every
joint supplies, according to the effective
working by which every part does its share,
causes growth of the body for the edifying
of itself in love.* —Ephesians 4:15-16

Liver congestion from poor diet choices, including lymph-plugging dairy, results in acne and other skin lesions. Sugar and dairy consumption can create referred pain to the left shoulder blade and neck. Constipation can lead to headaches. Signs of a stressed thyroid are thinning hair and yellow teeth.

FASTING

Fasting promotes digestive tract rest. I have fasted with vegetable broth and a plant-based protein supplement for up to two weeks. An easily digested protein will help prevent muscle breakdown. Generally it may take up to 24 hours for your body to adjust without hunger pains. Make sure you drink plenty of water. You may have a caffeine or sugar withdrawal headache; blood vessels will be pounding. You can lose up to 14 pounds in two weeks. Limit food choices to fruit and vegetables for three days for your first fast.

Day 214

RAISING BRAN

Eat more whole grains, especially bran cereals that are high in fiber (at least five grams per serving). They're usually a richer source of fiber than bran muffins, wheat bran bread, oat bran bread, or whole-wheat bread.

HEALTHY OILS

Your body needs oil and fat to operate at peak performance; low-fat, fat-free foods leave your body in a deficient state. Focus on balancing your meals to include items prepared with olive oil, which can be heated to moderate temperatures. Flax oil, a common but deficient oil in our culture, promotes heart and brain health. Flax oil actively reduces pain and should not be heated. Start taking a quality, organic flax oil product today. A logical amount is one tablespoon per 100 pounds of body weight. Do not heat flax oil.

NECESSARY SUPPLEMENTS

Optimal oil function and physiology are necessary for cell function. You may be unknowingly suffering from hormonal challenges, including hot flashes, dry skin, fatigue, and depression because you are using the inappropriate oil for your body. We use a simple blood test to assess our patients' levels and commonly notice a lack of Omega 3 oils, low zinc levels, and too much Omega 6 and trans fat. You can go to www.druglessdoctor.com for details on how you can receive a kit sent directly to your home to be forwarded on to a lab.

TIME FOR AN OIL CHANGE

"…How long will you mourn for Saul, seeing I have rejected him from reigning over Israel? Fill your horn with oil, and go…". —FIRST SAMUEL 16:1

Your body requires oil to function. There are two critical oils your body cannot make on its own, called essential fatty acids. Clinical-based evidence from diet journaling suggests we get more than enough of the Omega 6 essential fats from snack foods. Even supposedly "healthy" expeller pressed oils such as safflower and sunflower can create an imbalance when too much is consumed.

HEALTHY OLIVE OIL

Olive oil is great on salads, breads, and for sautéing, and it should be used in a rotation of oil choices. I strongly encourage flax oil—which needs to be refrigerated, never heated, and is an excellent source of Omega 3 fats. Flax oil is not commonly used in most meal planning. One tablespoon daily per 100 pounds is a good place to start. Put it on salads, breads, potatoes, rice, or straight up. Omega 6-rich safflower, sunflower, primrose, borage, and black currant oils can be transformed into painful arachidonic acid when consumed consistently. Use olive oil and flax oil, in addition to other healthy oils.

FLAX SEED OIL

Flax seeds are pressed oil, one of the two essential oils needed for the body to thrive. Flax, also called linseed oil, goes through steps to make two other fats called DHA or EPA. EPA is a fat that is used by the body to help promote heart and blood vessel health. DHA is important to support brain and nervous system health. I have seen patients with depression, headaches, anxiety, ADHD, and other conditions improve by consuming one tablespoon of flax oil per 100 pounds of body weight. This is a winner of a supplement!

HUMAN-MADE FAT VERSUS GOD-MADE FAT

*Bring your father and your households
and come to me; I will give you the best
of the land of Egypt, and you will eat
the fat of the land.* —GENESIS 45:18

Focus on oils in nature. Olive oil, which can be heated, and flax oil, which should not be heated, are affordable, healthy oils. I have incorporated coconut oil in our practice for patients who want to heat an oil at higher temperature without using human-made trans fats. Ultimately, my advice is to avoid fried foods and to never use trans fat, hydrogenated, or partially hydrogenated fat. Stay away from any human-made oil, regardless of how safe the research says it is.

PETER'S FISH

...go to the sea, cast in a hook, and take the fish that comes up first.... —MATTHEW 17:27

Peter and John must have consumed fish regularly since that was their livelihood. Fish is an excellent source of DHA fat and protein for brain food. Broiled fish or covered and baked fish on the grill is an excellent method of preparing fish dishes. A dash of lemon and fresh herbs add flavor. Avoid deep-fried fish at all costs and do not eat raw fish. Parasite eggs that are microscopic in size can grow into parasites over 40 feet long. Parasites eat first and afterward they release toxic excrements. They leave you the leftovers—at best. Add broiled or baked ocean fish to your diet rotation. Outside grilling is my favorite!

PASS THE OLIVE OIL

...you shall tread the olives.... —MICAH 6:15

The Mediterranean diet, which includes olives and simple complex foods, promotes heart health. Cholesterol levels are similar between the Mediterranean diet and the typical Western plan; however, there are one-third less hospitalizations for heart disease in the Mediterranean diet. Focus more on fresh fruits, nuts, legumes, and whole foods versus Danish, cookies, fries, and convenience, packaged items.

HAVE A PLAN

Having no plan is a plan to fail. Start planning Mediterranean-style foods in your meals. Be sure to include fresh vegetables, fruit, and organic chicken or turkey. To save money, buy the poultry on sale and freeze it in amounts your family will eat. Try sautéing a variety of vegetables in olive oil—only a spritz—and add Celtic Sea Salt and herbs. Vegetables in olive oil complement any meal. Use olive oil, basil, and a freshly squeezed lemon wedge as a salad dressing on your mixed greens.

BUTTER OR MARGARINE?

*The words of his mouth were smoother
than butter....* —PSALM 55:21

Is butter better than margarine? Margarine is a human-made toxic substance that promotes the disease it was supposed to help. So much for that. Butter is a neutral fat, not good and not bad. It is not necessary and in excess is dangerous. Butter is useful for frying because it tolerates high heat and is easy to digest. You can make butter better by adding high oleic safflower or sunflower oil to it and mixing them together for heating. To spread on breads, add flax oil to butter for a flavorful nutty twist.

BENEFITS OF BUTTER

Butter is low in the essential fatty acids and has high levels of other fats that compete with flax. One pound of butter does contain one gram of cholesterol, which may be an issue for some who have high cholesterol affected by diet. Butter does not have all the factors in itself to be properly metabolized, and it does have a small amount of natural trans fat. Always choose God-made versus human-made food items.

Day 226

FAT CRAVING SNACK FOOD?

So he called the name of that place Kibroth Hattaavah, because there they buried the people who had yielded to craving. —NUMBERS 11:34

I believe that people crave food unknowingly. The public is attracted to the preservatives, taste enhancers, and nitrates. The body literally has an endorphin reaction high from the excitotoxin stimulation. Trans fats, partially and totally hydrogenated, are in salty, addictive snack foods. Americans consume approximately 25 to 30 pounds of snacks per year. Read labels and avoid items containing trans fat. A "low fat" label may actually be a red flag for trans fat or other toxic human-made fat substitutes.

TRANS FAT

Trans fat is vegetable oil that has been heated and had hydrogen added. This fat was developed in volume to lower cholesterol levels, but in actuality it raises the LDL cholesterol and lowers the HDL cholesterol. You cannot fool Mother Nature. Trans fat is incorporated into cell membranes causing the cells to become hardened. The metabolism of other fat pathways are sabotaged with trans fat snack food consumption for up to 102 days. ADHD, depression, Alzheimer's, and pain can all result because of trans fat. But don't overdo safflower or sunflower oil for snacks either. Even though they are not trans fat and are healthier, over-consuming these oils can result in pain.

HAND PAIN

Hand and finger pain can be disabling. A common condition I frequently assist is "trigger finger." The tendons located on the palm aspect of your hand can become irritated with small stress centers. This is normally a result of poor fat metabolism due to a whole food B6 deficiency. The body will send what feels like a bean substance as a healing mechanism. This growth can actually get trapped, preventing your finger from relaxing. The result is a snap noise, and it is painful.

TRIGGER FINGERS

Trigger fingers are a symptom of a deeper problem, which is poor metabolism of a fat-like substance for pain relief called Prostaglandin 3. You can actually get tendonitis in other areas beside the finger, elbow, wrist, shoulder, hip, ankle, or toe. Consume one tablespoon of flax daily per 100 pounds and add a whole food B6 to your supplement protocol, 150 milligrams daily. Eliminate trans or partially hydrogenated fat from your diet. They stop the good Prostaglandin, PG-3, production.

Day 230

INFUSE YOUR OLIVE OIL

*For the Lord your God is bringing you into
a good land,…a land of wheat and barley, of
vines and fig trees and pomegranates, a land
of olive oil and honey;* —DEUTERONOMY 8:7-8

Herbs are discussed from the very beginning of creation. We use herbs in our home year round. My suggestion is go to your health food store and purchase single containers of herbs, one per week. Add them to your salads. Add your favorite herb to the food you prepare near the end of cooking. Adding herbs too soon may deplete the essence due to the warming process. I enjoy basil, dill, parsley, thyme, oregano, and chives.

INFUSED OLIVE OIL

Periodically I purchase a gallon of olive oil and add a variety of my favorite herbs and sun dried tomatoes to the container. The herbs are absorbed by the oil for three weeks. I pour off the oil into dark, rubber-sealed bottles using a fine sieve or strainer and store the bottles in a dark, cool cupboard or pantry. You will passionately fall in love with the enriched flavor. Olive oil is an excellent source of fat that is good for you. Sauté your favorite vegetables with olive oil over moderate heat. My motto: If Jesus used it, which I am sure He did, so can I.

DEPRESSION IS SERIOUS

*Truly the light is sweet, and it is
pleasant for the eyes to behold the
sun;* —ECCLESIASTES 11:7

It is my experience that depression is common among individuals who live in dreary, lack-of-sunshine climates. The ability to be outside in the sun impacts your emotional health. Sun helps the emotions by facilitating the movement of fat and minerals, all needed for brain health. Those who live in cloud-covered areas should increase their flax oil during winter months, especially if they have dry, flaky skin. Add liquid sunshine, flax oil, to your diet, one tablespoon per 100 pounds of body weight.

BE A NUT

Moreover the word of the Lord came to me, saying, "Jeremiah, what do you see?" And I said, "I see a branch of an almond tree." Then the Lord said to me, "You have seen well, for I am ready to perform My word." —JEREMIAH 1:11-12

Nuts are an excellent source of protein and good fat. I generally prepare a small container of raw nuts daily to eat midmorning or afternoon. Protein is to the body what a log is to fire—a slow-burning source of fuel. Raw nuts provide a steady blood sugar response and reduce hunger. Add nuts to your breakfast routine, quinoa, grits, non-gluten, or gluten cereals. I generally eat raw cashews, almonds, and walnuts.

THE BENEFIT OF NUTS

Walnuts are not a common "health food" topic, but they are a super source of Omega 3 fat. Almonds are a neutral nut, not acidic or alkaline and they add calcium to the system. I also enjoy sesame seeds, which are an excellent source of calcium, and sunflower seeds. Sprinkle the seeds on any item you like. Pumpkin seeds are a good source of zinc. Peanuts are not nuts; they are legumes and can create problems for some. Beware that red or white pistachios are generally overcooked and can be rancid.

STOP PAIN

Before them the people writhe in pain; all faces are drained of color. —JOEL 2:6

Relentless pain can stop the best of anyone in their tracks. What you eat either promotes or suppresses fat tissue-like hormones in your body. Decrease pain by eating flax oil, walnuts, greens, and deepwater ocean fish. Avoid eating red meat, dairy, and shellfish, which can increase pain. Add flax (one tablespoon per 100 pounds daily), with alfalfa tablets (four to six daily).

ESSENTIAL OILS

Our body uses oil to make hormones, cell membranes, energy, and it even gives taste to food. Dry skin, especially in the winter, is a blinking red light that you need oil. Fat and oil consumption can be confusing. An excellent oil source for salad dressings and sautéing is olive oil. Olive oil, from an organic source, first pressed without heat or chemical extraction, is an excellent choice. I do not recommend a low-fat diet. Fat is needed for function in all organs, but don't overdo it. Flax oil on salad is an excellent healthy habit. Try using organic coconut oil on bread or toast, it is an excellent alternative for butter.

CAN OIL BE SOFT?

...His words were softer than oil.... —PSALM 55:21

Cell membranes in the body are made up of different types of fats, oil, and cholesterol. Saturated fat is firm, or hard, at room temperature and creates hardness in the walls of blood vessels. You can improve the softness of blood vessel walls by using flax or olive oil. Consume one tablespoon of organic flax oil daily. This is equivalent to approximately twelve capsules.

DANDRUFF—HEAD SKIN ITCH

If a man or woman has a sore [or skin itch] *on the head....* —LEVITICUS 13:29

Inflammation of the scalp and head can be quite annoying. Billions of dollars are spent each year on shampoos designed to control exfoliation of skin on top of the head. Watch for chemicals that you are applying to your brain, which is adjacent to the skull. The scalp and tissues around the head and face are rich with blood vessels. Sodium lauryl sulfate, a common toxic ingredient, is going to be absorbed, evenslightly, and over time there will be an accumulation, causing liver congestion.

TREATING DANDRUFF

I treat most patients with dandruff, seborrhea, and eczema with a balance of oils. The oils should have a combination of the Omega 6 and Omega 3 fats. Generally patients are deficient in the Omega 3 fats such as flax oil. For whatever reason, dandruff responds more effectively to a product we use called BioOmega with a combination of Omega 3 oils. Skin inflammation, just as other body inflammations, responds with the right oil. Read product ingredient labels on all lotions you apply to your skin. Avoid sodium lauryl sulfate. One tablespoon of a balance of Omega 6 and 3 oils per 100 pounds of body weight will heal dry skin challenges.

AVOID PAIN

Yet, I am glad now, not because you were pained, but because you were pained into repentance [and so turned back to God];
—SECOND CORINTHIANS 7:9
AMPLIFIED BIBLE

Pain is a sign of inflammation. First, the leading cause of pain is the improper metabolism of a tissue fat hormone called Prostaglandin 3, or PG3. PG3 production is interrupted by lack of vitamins and minerals, especially B vitamins, zinc, and magnesium. Second, the leading factor depleting these important ingredients is stress and sugar. What should you do? Delete sugar from your diet, reduce stress (exercise helps), and take PG3-promoting flax oil.

Day 241

FEELING STRESSED?

You will keep in perfect peace all who trust in you, all whose thoughts are fixed on you!
—Isaiah 26:3 New Living Translation

It may surprise you to learn that not all stress is bad. In fact, some stress is very beneficial. What determines whether it is good or bad is how much stress you are under. A little stress can be good. Today we have people yelling "fire" at us constantly. Over time, the body wears down, and you slip into the resistance stage. Frequent alarms precipitate chronic illness. Focus on modifying the stress factors. Add adrenal tissue support, whole foods, pantothenic acid, and vitamin C to your life. Do not over-commit to responsibilities.

Day 242

IODINE

Iodine supplementation is critically important today for optimal function for all the cells in the body. Iodine is necessary not only for thyroid utilization; it is also used and needed by the ovaries, breasts, and testes in men. There is a group of elements in the iodine or halide family called bromine, fluorine, and chlorine. These three compete with iodine, often disrupting the position of iodine at the cellular level. We live in a very toxic environment, with an abundance of chlorine when we shower and swim, fluorine when we drink water or brush our teeth, and bromine in white bread and sports drinks. Supplement iodine in your diet to combat these toxins.

ABSORBABLE CALCIUM

But where can wisdom be found? And where is the place of understanding?...No mention shall be made of coral or quartz, for the price of wisdom is above rubies. —JOB 28:12,18

Calcium is a foundation mineral in the framework of our bone structure. The skeletal system is the attachment for tendons, ligaments, and muscles. Calcium is needed by the bony framework like limestone in concrete. Focus on calcium that is easily absorbed. I encourage my female patients to take flax oil and to participate in resistance exercises, as well as avoid sugar and soda. Remember, sunshine helps calcium absorption.

Day 244

VARICOSE VEINS

Varicose veins, common in men and women with congested livers, can create cosmetic and physical issues. Pregnancy, also a stress on the female liver, can cause varicose or spider veins. Another reason for varicose veins is a deficiency of whole food B vitamins. Your body needs B vitamins to process estrogen. Eat beets daily and take your whole food B vitamins.

SNACKING ON NUTS

It's worth adding small servings of nuts to your diet; just keep in mind that they are calorie-dense, so you can't eat them without removing something else. (The study's authors recommend deleting some refined grains and red meat.) There is 150 to 185 calories in a one-ounce serving of dry roasted nuts. That's just twenty-two almonds or fourteen walnut halves.

BLESSED IS THE WOMB

...Blessed is the womb that bore
You.... —LUKE 11:27

The value of a healthy womb is price-
less. Fibroids and heavy menstrual flow
are very common in our toxic society. Why
does a toxic environment impact the uterus?
Because estrogen clearing is delayed in the
liver. Your liver processes estrogen with the
help of quality B vitamins. Avoiding sugar,
trans fat, alcohol, and even some prescription
medications will go a long way to improving
uterus health and entire body health.

EXTREME MENSTRUAL FLOW

If a woman has a discharge of blood many days, other than at the time of her customary impurity, or if it runs beyond her usual time.... —LEVITICUS 15:25

The leading cause of heavy or extensive menstrual flow is poor diet choices and stress. Stress depletes the body of badly needed whole food B vitamins that are necessary to process estrogen. The liver is programmed to create chemicals to handle the additional emotional load. Ladies, before deciding to have a hysterectomy, my suggestion is to first focus on a detoxification program and lifestyle pattern change.

Day 248

PREVENTING OSTEOPOROSIS

Osteoporosis, or loss of calcium from bone, creates a state of fragility. When was the last time you saw an adult cow eating cottage cheese, milk, or ice cream? Cows eat hay, grass, and alfalfa for their sources of calcium. Excellent sources of calcium for you include sesame seeds, mixed greens, almonds, and alfalfa.

SEASONAL EMOTIONS

For the day of the Lord...is at hand: a day of darkness and gloominess, a day of clouds and thick darkness.... —JOEL 2:1-2

Some people become more depressed in the winter months when the days are shorter and darker. Exercise daily and enjoy the sunshine whenever possible. The pineal gland in your brain is affected by sunlight. I discourage sunglasses. They block precious sunlight to your retina. Increase potassium for adrenal support so your eyes will be less bothered by light. Cucumbers and alfalfa are excellent sources of potassium.

VITAMIN D IS FREE

The sun also rises, and the sun goes down, and hastens to the place where it arose. —ECCLESIASTES 1:5

The Lord put the sun in the sky for a purpose. One of the roles of the sun is to convert the cholesterol in your skin to vitamin D. Vitamin D is critical for optimal calcium absorption. My advice to patients is to enjoy the morning and evening sun. Think of sun as a natural cholesterol-lowering medication and an osteoporosis supplement.

BE FRUITFUL AND MULTIPLY

Then God blessed them, and God said to them, "Be fruitful and multiply...." —GENESIS 1:28

Pregnancy is not always easily possible for individuals with low thyroid gland function. Progesterone is often deficient in individuals who are not capable of carrying a child full term. Also, the antinutrient—sugar—sabotages the body from properly carrying out its desire to reproduce itself. Add organic kelp tablets, deep ocean fish, and alfalfa sprouts or tablets to feed the thyroid iodine.

"Wait Until You Have Weaned Him"

...Then the woman stayed and nursed her son until she had weaned him. —First Samuel 1:23

There are natural laws and principles that do not change. God designed females' breasts to feed their offspring. Human breast milk has the factors in it to promote a strong immune system. Children who are bottle fed with human-made formulas often have allergies. Soy-based formulas can deplete the body of zinc and calcium. Instead, breast-feed your children so they can get a head start with a healthy immune system.

EASILY BRUISED

Broken blood vessels result in blood escaping into tissue, leading to bruising. Bruising is not uncommon in women with heavy menstrual flow, and heavy menstrual flow generally occurs with high estrogen. Clean up your choices—no sugar, no trans fat. Aspirin use, which disrupts your body from working properly, creates fragile blood cells resulting in bruises. Use flax oil for pain and to keep blood cells moving freely. Have vitamin C-rich, colored bell peppers as a midmorning snack.

ESTHER'S BODY LOTION

*Each young woman's turn came to go in
to King Ahasuerus after she had completed
twelve months' preparation, according to
the regulations for the women, for thus were
the days of their preparation apportioned:
six months with oil of myrrh, and six
months with perfumes and preparations
for beautifying women.* —ESTHER 2:12

I want you to be aware of what you put
in and on your body. What you apply
is absorbed through the skin and travels
through the lymphatic system and is processed in the liver. Today lotions and body
applications may create a toxic state.

TOXIC COSMETICS

Become a label reader. Sodium lauryl sulfate (SLS) and sodium laureth sulfate (SLES) are major ingredients in cosmetics, toothpaste, and 90 percent of all shampoos and products that foam. They have been described as "dangerous beauty." Read all labels of products that you apply to your skin. They may be causing chronic pain, allergies, skin irritations, and depression.

TROUBLESHOOTING BELLY PAIN

*And He said to them, "What kind
of conversation is this that you
have with one another as you walk
and are sad?"* —LUKE 24:17

It is possible that, after all other logical causes of stomach pain have been ruled out, emotional sadness and distress may, in fact, be causing your pain. The depth of your breathing is restricted when your diaphragm is not fully relaxing or contracting. The diaphragm shares an attachment with another muscle called the psoas, which is centered in the lower belly. When you have emotional sadness, you may experience pain, especially slightly off to the right upper quadrant. A skilled massage therapist can help relax the imbalance.

SPEND TIME WITH YOUR FAMILY

Men need to spend time with their families. Plan time to be with your immediate family daily. Turn off the media and game center for 21 days and concentrate on your family. Start with a minimum of ten minutes daily for one week and then work up to thirty minutes—find one activity all can agree on. From Day 15 on, go for a walk together or ride or drive—look at the stars, read a book out loud to each other. I continue to have regular time with my sons and wife every day. Set up a time and commit to each other.

JACOB'S HIP

Now when He saw that he did not prevail against him, He touched the socket of his hip; and the socket of Jacob's hip was out of joint as He wrestled with him. —GENESIS 32:25

A posture imbalance, with weight being carried on one side more than the other because of trauma or injury, can cause one hip to wear out before the other. Obesity creates enormous additional stress for the hips. Have an appropriate assessment for hip and pelvis pain including standing postural X-rays. Look at heel wear on your shoes. Uneven wear may indicate pelvic hip imbalance.

BREATHE DEEPLY

And the Lord God formed man of the dust of the ground, and breathed into his nostrils the breath of life; and man became a living being. —GENESIS 2:7

Oxygen is essential for life. Deep breathing belly exercises strengthen the abdominal tissues responsible for lung expansion. Taking a few deep breaths periodically is like giving your brain a blast of unexpected oxygen. Your neurons will celebrate. Try it, your brain will thank you.

BREATHING, IT'S IMPORTANT

Breathe in through your nose and determine which nostril is not functioning at full capacity. Plug the one with the most intake and breathe in the nostril that was functioning less. Also, erect postural alignment expands the lung's ability to take in more oxygen for fuel. Stand and take ten deep breaths.

MINERAL DEFICIENCIES

People who have low energy and memory loss often have a zinc deficiency. Zinc is needed to make insulin, a factor needed for carbohydrate metabolism. Copper is often elevated in individuals with a low zinc level. When copper is elevated in females, I also see high estrogen levels with associated symptoms of PMS—heavy menstrual flow and tender breast tissue. Low zinc also affects the male prostate.

CHECKING FOR DEFICIENCIES

Hair mineral tissue analysis is a logical evaluation of body function. Reduce wheat and soy, as they deplete zinc. Raw pumpkin seeds are an excellent source of zinc.

FEET AND TOE HEALTH

Foot and toe health is a snapshot of whole body function. Pain on the inside of the heels may indicate prostate issues. When you have a full body yeast problem, it can result in fungus growth under all the nails. Fungus on the toes creates green coloration—this is serious.

YEAST LOVES SUGAR

Yeast and fungus grow in a sweet environment. We strongly encourage our patients to avoid baked goods with yeast, sweet fruits, and sugar. Full body yeast and fungus also may cause jockstrap itch in men. Focus on foods with low sugar, greens, and protein. Avoid fruit juices.

DON'T SIT STILL

If you're overweight, keep moving. Walk rather than ride. Don't sit when you can stand, and keep moving when you have to sit. Move to the music from your car radio. Lift weights or do sit-ups while you watch TV, and so forth.

CHILDREN ARE A REWARD FROM THE LORD

Children are a gift from the Lord;
they are a reward from him. —PSALM
127:3 NEW LIVING TRANSLATION

Do you want happy, healthy children? Speak happy, healthy, uplifting words. Do not make your children live your dreams. They have dreams of their own. Take short trips together when you don't have the budget for longer vacations, such as weekend college football games, fishing outings, the zoo, ball games, museums, plays, musicals, high school events, or play soccer. There is a huge list of events to match all schedules and budgets.

Upon This Rock

*I also say to you that you are Peter,
and on this rock I will build My
church....* —Matthew 16:18

Assimilating rock minerals is necessary for proper body function. I have noticed, especially in men, a mineral consumption and absorption issue resulting in bowed legs. An excellent source of calcium includes (beside rock) sesame seeds and almonds. Alfalfa sprouts and Celtic Sea Salt are also great sources of minerals.

HAIR LOSS AND LOW THYROID

For every head shall be bald....
—JEREMIAH 48:37

Body signals, including the number of hairs on your head (whether male or female) are windows to how the inside is functioning. A common cause of hair loss, especially seen in females, is a low thyroid. Additional common symptoms include cold hands and feet, headaches in the morning that diminish as the day goes on, constipation, fatigue, wide-spaced teeth, and thin, sparse hair.

SAFELY EATING WILD GAME

If you are a hunter and you consume wild game like venison, squirrel, or rabbit, here's a tip. Soak your meat in a citric seed extract to neutralize any "unfriendly" organisms. Cook your meat thoroughly. Parasites are easily transmitted in undercooked food. Wild game has the potential to have an abundance of parasites. This is one of several reasons why commercially prepared animals are treated with antibiotics.

YOUR FUEL PUMP—THE ADRENAL GLAND

The adrenal gland is your "Fight or Flight" escape backup—it is in a constant state of exhaustion for most Westerners. The adrenals are fatigued from burning the candle at both ends and eating refined carbohydrates such as cookies, cakes, pasta, and sweet fruits. This is a very important gland that needs support to rebuild. Take time to rest between projects. The hours you spend in bed sleeping before midnight are essential for optimal health.

CUT OFF MY HEADACHE

Headaches can be so painful that people have been known to pound their heads on a wall to relieve the head pain. Morning headaches that go away as the day progresses may be caused by a low functioning thyroid gland. To prevent morning headaches, do not eat fruit or sweets at night.

SLOW TO ANGER

He who is slow to anger is better than the mighty, and he who rules his spirit than he who takes a city. —PROVERBS 16:32

Anger is an explosive emotion. Anger requires the liver to work harder. Patients with emotional stress, including anger, tend to have more liver-related symptoms of disease including pain, gallbladder distress, arthritis, and even cancer. Make it a priority to eat in an environment of peace, often at home with loved ones.

GOUT

If the foot should say, "Because I am not a hand, I am not of the body," is it therefore not of the body? —FIRST CORINTHIANS 12:15

Gout is a common type of arthritis where there is too much uric acid in the blood, tissues, and urine. Uric acid is the end product of a food group called purines (pork and organ meats). The crystals can be sharp, which create pain, especially common in the big toe due to pressure in walking. Gout has been called the "rich man's disease" since it has been associated with too much rich food and alcohol.

KEEPING YOUR KIDNEYS CLEAN

I encourage my patients to eat parsley with each meal. Parsley is a natural cleanser for kidney function. Men appear to have more "gout" attacks than women. From my experience, the kidneys kick in as the "second liver." When the liver is stressed, the overflow of toxins is placed on kidney function. Avoid pork, hot dogs, sausage, and alcohol. Clean machines work better. Turkey bacon makes a great BLT with safflower oil mayonnaise.

MINERALS IN YOUR HAIR

Your body requires additional minerals when stressed. Your body does not need hair on your head to survive. The minerals normally stored in the hair are used by the body as cellular spark plugs for chemical reactions to keep the engine going. The adrenal gland needs to be supported. Supplement your diet with mineral-rich foods like alfalfa and Celtic Sea Salt. Avoid mineral-depleting sugar.

Eat Lean, Grass Fed, Organic Beef

Look for beef from an organic source. Antibiotics, growth hormones, and steroids are clipped onto the ears of cows in commercial farms. The additives enter the tissue of the coat and settle in highest concentration in fat. Cows raised on grass (versus grain) on an open range where they can walk around have more health benefits. You can receive good fat from beef.

DETECTIVE WORK

*And it will become fine dust in all the land of Egypt, and it will cause **boils that break out** in sores on man and beast....* —EXODUS 9:9

One of the top devastating conditions affecting modern people is Type II diabetes. Diabetic boils erupt because bacteria thrive in a high blood sugar environment. The significant point is that the condition is preventable. Lose weight. This will take stress off the pancreas. Eating raw, whole food loaded with enzymes will take stress off the pancreas. Avoid processed food.

OPTIMAL HEALTH FOR CHILDREN

Jesus learned by example from His parents. What you do is what your children will do. Spend time with your children. Make life fun. Go to their events and cheer them on! Create a loving, peaceful home environment. Children have real pain. Children love to be held and comforted. Try cooking together on weekends. Always feed them food aimed at providing optimal health!

Day 279

FEED YOUR KIDS RIGHT

*The children of your people will live
in security. Their children's children
will thrive in your presence.* —PSALM
102:28 NEW LIVING TRANSLATION

What you feed your kids can overwork their livers, leading to liver stress even early in their lives. I really believe that breastfeeding is best. Goat's milk is a viable option. Avoid milk; it causes ear infections and allergies. Use almond, rice, or coconut milk.

HEALTHY FOODS, HEALTHY KIDS

Do not feed children solid food too soon. Avoid soda and hydrogenated fats. Soda pop depletes calcium, and the sodium benzoate can cause food allergies. Use almond butter for calcium. Purchase spelt flour bread, brown rice for a grain, and real oatmeal. Your children will eat what they see you eat. Eat healthy foods!

GROWING PAINS

...they ate their food with gladness and simplicity of heart, praising God and having favor with all the people. And the Lord added to the church daily those who were being saved. —ACTS 2:46-47

Growing pains in children are commonly caused by a functional low thyroid. Cold hands and feet are a common low thyroid body signal. Measure a child's armpit temperature first thing in the morning before the child gets out of bed. The temperature should be 97.8 or above. I suggest organic iodine, one daily, if below 97.8 degrees. Vegetables, kelp, and Celtic Sea Salt are also sources of iodine.

Day 282

A KOR OF SODA

The ordinance concerning oil, the bath
of oil, is one-tenth of a bath from a kor.
A kor is a homer or ten baths, for ten
baths are a homer. —EZEKIEL 45:14

The average American consumes over a kor of soft drinks (soda) per year. A kor is a biblical measure of fifty-plus gallons. That's a lot of soda. Teenage males consume the most—as many as four to six twelve-ounce containers daily. Soda is not water and is not to be counted as part of your daily water intake. Diet soda, regardless of your reason to drink it, causes enormous toxic stress to the liver.

WATCH YOUR COMPANY

Do not be deceived: "Evil company corrupts good habits." —FIRST CORINTHIANS 15:33

Once you have made a decision to alter your health lifestyle, seek out individuals with similar desires. Look at what people who didn't agree with Jesus did to Him. Jealousy, envy, and strife may occur because many may not like the changes you are making. This happens in my practice frequently. Let your light of improved health, weight loss, reduced pain, and emotional stability shine in the darkness.

PREPARE FOR TEMPTATION

People often resist change. Addiction to food and habits are perceived to be difficult to break. Individuals who crave milk may need fat, protein, and calcium. I tell patients to increase flax, chicken, turkey, beans, and sesame seeds to combat food cravings and addictions.

ADDICTED TO SUGAR

Sugar addictions are exceedingly common. Chromium is a mineral that is often deficient in people with sugar cravings, which you may need to supplement into your diet. Family members can prove to be challenging when you are trying to change. You can't change them; use your God-given discipline to say, "No thank you." Have alternatives to processed "goodies" on hand when you are confronted with a treat.

WHAT'S HOT?

*And standing over her, He rebuked the
fever, and it left her; and immediately she
got up....* —LUKE 4:39 AMPLIFIED BIBLE

Having an elevated temperature is often
helpful to the body. This is a defense
mechanism of the body acting to destroy
harmful microbes. A temperature above 102
degrees in adults or 103 degrees in children
should be monitored by your healthcare
provider. You should be checked by your
healthcare provider if you have a headache,
swollen glands, a rash, vomiting, or pain in
the abdomen accompanied by a fever.

CHILDREN'S HEALTH

*Blessed is the man who fears the Lord.
...His descendants will be mighty
on earth....* —PSALM 112:1-2

Baby oil is 100 percent mineral oil. This substance is a commonly used petroleum ingredient that coats the skin just like what is used in plastic wrap. The skin's natural immune barrier is disrupted as this plastic coating inhibits its ability to breathe and absorb moisture and nutrition. This can promote acne and other disorders.

Day 288

TOXIC ABSORPTION

What you apply to your skin is easily absorbed through the lymph channels. Toxic accumulation occurs over time. Observe the number of brown marks on your teens. They increase in number as the liver is overloaded with fries, soda, and junk food. Read ingredient labels. What is applied to the skin—including self-tanner pigments and sprays—needs to be processed and incorporated into the cells or eliminated. Why overwork the system?

YOU WILL BE KNOWN BY YOUR FRUIT

For if the firstfruit is holy, the lump is also holy; and if the root is holy, so are the branches. —ROMANS 11:16

The quality of fruit produced by a plant or tree is directly related to the health of the tree, the water, soil contents, and the sunshine or lack of it. Your daily habit patterns create the state of the environment and fruit in your life. A common eating pattern is soda consumption. Soda is loaded with ingredients that stress the liver and nervous system. Sodium benzoate, which is used as a preservative, can be a cause of chronic allergies and ADHD or ADD.

HEALTHY CHOICES, HEALTHY FAMILIES

Grazing on partially hydrogenated snack foods impairs the body's ability to make essential brain fat. You may need to tend to your own garden more effectively. Spend time creating patterns that promote life for you and your family.

SUPERSIZE ME!

Whoever keeps the law is a discerning son, but a companion of gluttons shames his father. —PROVERBS 28:7

Develop new life patterns for you and your family. It is a matter of life and death. Plan your meals. Purchase an insulator bag with blue ice for travel. Almond butter and jelly travel well.

Day 292

CHEEK TO CHEEK

They gape at me with their mouth, they strike me reproachfully on the cheek.... —JOB 16:10

Cheek health and integrity speak a book to an astute detective. Large facial pores are a sign of low zinc. Zinc can be depleted with wheat and soy consumption. Small blood vessels on the cheeks and nose may be a sign of elevated estrogen levels in females, suggesting a need for whole food B vitamins to process elevated estrogen levels. Small skin tabs and brown moles or nevi also suggest liver congestion. Eat grated raw or baked organic beets.

Skin Health

Small multiple "blackheads" suggest poor liver processing of fats and oils. Freckles showing up on the front cheeks by the nose bridge at about eight to twelve years old also suggest liver congestion with high copper and low zinc. Consuming dairy, especially for teens, congests the lymph system, resulting in facial acne. Substitute raw almonds and sesame seeds for calcium in teens with milk-induced acne.

UPRIGHT POSTURE

...When [Saul] stood among the people, he was taller than any of the people from his shoulders upward. —FIRST SAMUEL 10:23

Maintaining erect posture requires energy. I instruct my patients to make a conscious effort to stand erect. Correct posture, with the shoulders gently rolled back, will increase the expansion of lung tissue. Increased chest capacity increases oxygen in the system promoting internal health with more energy, clearer thinking, and even reduced sickness. Focus on a conscious awareness to stand erect.

CHILDREN

The righteous man walks in his integrity; his children are blessed after him. —PROVERBS 20:7

My wife and I established a regular pattern with our children. We spent our evenings reading and playing. Every night we were on our knees praying. We read Bible stories and simple books. On Saturdays, I made a special breakfast or we went out. Sunday was church and grandparents day. We established a regular pattern every day. My sons always knew when dad was home. Spend time with your family. You only have them for a short time. Plan an event today.

HYPERACTIVITY AND HEALTH

Eliminating trans fat is the leading factor for reducing ADHD symptoms. Trans fat sabotages your body from making DHA, the long-chain fat needed for brain health. Unfortunately trans fat or partially hydrogenated fat is everywhere. Depression responds to the same supplement protocol as ADHD. Avoid trans fat, take one salmon capsule per night for eighteen nights. Add six whole food B vitamins daily. Take B6, 150 milligrams daily; alfalfa tablets, six daily for a multiple nutrient mineral source; and finally, one tablespoon of flax per 100 pounds of body weight.

TEACH YOUR CHILDREN THIS!

You shall love the Lord your God with all your heart, with all your soul, and with all your strength. ...You shall teach them diligently to your children, and shall talk of them when you sit in your house.... —DEUTERONOMY 6:5,7

Is God in your family's life? Do you speak about the blessings of the Lord in your life? Our family time included reading Bible stories to our children out loud, especially from the Book of Proverbs. We pray before each meal, a sincere prayer time. Attending church service on Sunday and during the week creates an atmosphere of godliness. Speak loving comments in your meal prayer time and conversation with the children in your life.

ALMOND BUTTER

*How is it you do not understand that I
did not speak to you concerning bread?—*
BUT TO BEWARE OF THE LEAVEN
[yeast] *of the Pharisees and Sadducees*
[peanuts]. —Matthew 16:11

My experience suggests that chronic sinus inflammation, allergies, headaches, and nasal congestion can be directly impacted by the amount of peanuts a person eats. Peanuts have a mold or yeast as part of their structure. This mold is toxic, especially over time with regular consumption. Replace peanut butter with almond butter. Almonds are a quality source of calcium and are neutral in pH, being neither acid nor alkaline. Sliced almonds also add flavor to any stir-fry meal.

WITHOUT A BLEMISH

Your lamb shall be without blemish.... —EXODUS 12:5

How can you reduce physical blemishes and skin eruptions? What about the ones that seem to appear without cause on the left cheek? Chronic left cheek blemishes are precipitated by liver congestion and adrenal gland stress. Why left? Liver and pancreas stress nearly always refer to the left neck, shoulder, and face, resulting in various signs and symptoms. Cleaning up your diet by minimizing sugar alone will reduce the blemishes by 30 to 40 percent in three months or less.

Day 300

FULL BODY BLEMISHES

Blemishes all over your body equate to more congestion and work for you to do. Eat carrots on your salad daily. They are an excellent source of vitamin A. Your body uses vitamin A for skin and liver restoration. Be patient. Do not have laser surgery for removing left cheek blemishes. They will return unless you clean your body from the inside out. Always remember that skin is used as part of the body detox system. Eat six baby carrots at your mid-afternoon break.

OPEN WIDE

*He has also broken my teeth with
gravel....* —LAMENTATIONS 3:16

Jesus talked about the eye as an entrance
to your spirit. I believe that the mouth is
the entrance to your physical self. The integrity
of teeth reveals much about the rest of
the body. The position, color, alignment,
and number of teeth affect your physical and
emotional health. Low thyroid function can
result in yellow teeth. Wide spaces between
the front teeth may be the result of a thyroid
that isn't working up to par.

SODA AND TEETH HEALTH

Soda consumption can create a phosphorous-calcium imbalance resulting in cavities when phosphorous is high or tartar when calcium is high. Loose teeth and a "pink toothbrush" can be a sign that more vitamin C from fruits and vegetables is required. Brush regularly and floss the teeth you want to keep—all of them! Limit, then eliminate, soda use. The phosphoric acid (substance that creates bubbles) depletes calcium.

TEACH YOUR KIDS RIGHT

Train up a child in the way he should go, and when he is old he will not depart from it. —PROVERBS 22:6

What are you speaking into your children? Spend time with your family. What do you eat? Are you overweight? Children will pick up your habits. Children of parents who smoke have access to cigarettes. Children mirror their environment. Make an effort to spend quality time with your children.

WARRANTY WORK

Clean machines work better. Water is the simplest, most cost-effective way to clean the body from the inside out. A suggestion during the next 21 days is to read the Book of Daniel and focus on what he did. Do you need a breakthrough in your life? For 21 days focus on eating fruits and veggies only. Be creative. Eat squash, steamed veggies, and fruit. Avoid coffee, tea, and soda. This is an excellent semiannual protocol.

NATURAL HEALING

"So he went to him and bandaged his wounds, pouring on oil and wine...." —LUKE 10:34

Does it seem like you are always sick? Do your health challenges linger? Why do some people get colds, bronchitis, and the flu and others do not? Stress depletes an important nutrient required for healing of wounds and colds. Zinc deficiencies can slow your body's ability to repair itself. Meat is an excellent source of zinc; pumpkin seeds and alfalfa are good plant sources of zinc. A body that heals slowly needs to be fed whole foods and detoxified of processed products.

THE FINEST OF WHEAT

"He would have fed them…the finest of wheat…." —PSALM 81:16

Our heavenly Father always wants His children to have the best. Wheat is an excellent source of B vitamins and vitamin E. The challenge today is that wheat has been stripped of all its nutrients. White bread without the bran and outer coverings is nutritionally a poor staple in comparison to biblical bread. I also see patients today, regardless of the source of wheat, who have some of their health issues caused by wheat sensitivities. I suggest that people should minimize wheat if they have chronic pain. Snoring may go away by eliminating wheat. Some food allergies are minimized by deleting wheat from your diet.

Day 307

DETOXIFICATION

We live in a time when air pollution is common worldwide. These toxins can congest the lymphatic system and the liver. Continuous breathing of petrochemicals is also challenging for the lungs and kidneys. We use the herb "larch gum" to cleanse the lymph system. Parsley in hot water or salads supports kidney function. Snip dandelion leaves for your salad to stimulate liver cleaning; and goldenseal used in limited amounts accelerates lung cleansing. Jesus came to die for our sin. He set us free from bondage. Set yourself free from the devastation of toxins. Keep your insides clean. Dandelion, goldenseal, fenugreek, and larch gum are all excellent God-given herbs for cleansing.

PROMOTING KNEE STRENGTH

Your words have upheld him who was stumbling, and you have strengthened the feeble knees. —JOB 4:4

Knee pain, like pain anywhere, can be annoying. You need your knees to move. Here are a couple of thoughts from my experience helping those "achy knees." Nagging pain on the inside of the knee can be from decay. Pain on the outside of the knee may oftentimes, ruling out an injury with an X-ray or MRI, be caused by gallbladder distress. Eat baked or raw beets. Beets help purify the liver and gallbladder partnership. Eighty percent of knee strength comes from muscles on the front of the thigh.

Day 309

READ MY LIPS

...an abomination to my lips. —PROVERBS 8:7

Every part of the body has a significant connection to every other part of the human machine. Cracks at the corner of the mouth, where the lips connect, are commonly caused by a deficiency of a whole food B vitamin called Riboflavin. A thin upper lip is also precipitated by a B vitamin deficiency. Cold sore eruptions nearly always point to a deficiency of easily assimilated calcium.

SUNSHINE AND CALCIUM

I often see travelers returning from a "sunshine" vacation erupt with cold sores due to the fact that sunshine depletes the body's reserves of calcium. Stress-related issues have a devastating toll on the body's use of calcium. Drinking water from a pure source bathes all the cells of the body including the lips. Add extra calcium citrate or lactate when you are spending long periods of time in the sun. Sea-sourced and digestive-aid-based calciums are challenging to absorb.

Day 311

CRUCIFEROUS VEGETABLES

He causes the grass to grow for the cattle, and vegetation for the service of man.... —PSALM 104:14

Broccoli, brussels sprouts, cabbage, and cauliflower fed to animals decreases cancer rates. The fiber from this food group assists the body in the elimination and binding of estrogen, reducing the risk for breast and ovarian cancer. Let food be your medicine.

EAT BROCCOLI

Chew everything thoroughly—and enjoy new levels of optimal health. You can also facilitate bowel movements by adding additional fiber to your diet. Patients who have a low functioning thyroid should limit cruciferous vegetables until thyroid function is improved. Rotate broccoli or cauliflower into your snack, salad, or supper regularly; rotate how you prepare the food items—raw, steamed, or sautéed.

THOUGHTS

Commit your works to the Lord, and your thoughts will be established. —PROVERBS 16:3

Do you cry without reason? Crying like this is typically a body signal of whole food B vitamin deficiencies. Relentless stress, which is common, depletes the body of B vitamins. You actually feel like you have raw nerves. The B vitamins are necessary ingredients for DNA, a protein needed for brain health and emotional function.

Day 314

GOOD GROUND

*"But other seed fell on good ground and yielded
a crop that sprang up, increased and produced:
some thirtyfold, some sixty, and some a
hundred." And He said to them, "He who has
ears to hear, let him hear!"* —MARK 4:8-9

Eating food sourced from mineral-rich organic soil is tastier and healthier than food from the over-farmed, pesticide- and herbicide-permeated conventional method. Toxic levels of aluminum and mercury are common with sluggish adrenal gland function. Calcium and magnesium are altered with thyroid function.

POSTURE WEIGHT TRAINING

You shall have a perfect and just weight, a perfect and just measure, that your days may be lengthened in the land which the Lord your God is giving you. —DEUTERONOMY 25:15

Weight training to tone muscle tissues only takes a few minutes, two or three times a week. I strongly suggest to all of my patients to obtain a large colored ball that you can fill with air. Lay on your back on the ball three to five minutes daily.

MEMORY BOOSTERS

Are not five sparrows sold for two copper coins? And not one of them is forgotten before God. —LUKE 12:6

I believe your memory is your most precious health asset. Alzheimer's and dementia are common today. Why? I believe the reasons include diet, stress, and bad effects from medication. The leading culprit is the depletion of key vitamins and minerals by consuming too much sugar. Your body needs minerals and vitamins to make a brain fat called DHA. Keep mineral levels high. Celtic Sea Salt, greens, and seeds are excellent mineral sources.

STIMULATE YOUR BRAIN

Keep your mind active with activities such as crossword puzzles and Scrabble. You need to exercise your mind like any other body tissue. Study and memorize Bible verses. We encourage flax oil, whole food B vitamins, and mixed greens for magnesium.

Day 318

WHAT CAUSES YOUR TEETH TO GRIND?

My flesh is caked with worms.... —JOB 7:5

Parasites can live in you an entire lifetime—if the environment is right. The most common consistent body signal is grinding teeth, especially at night. If you have a mouth guard for grinding, you may want to be checked for parasites. A high white blood cell, called eosinophil, on a complete blood count is a place to start but does not confirm.

CROSSWORDS AND ALZHEIMER'S

Reading newspapers or books, playing games like cards or checkers, doing crosswords or other puzzles, going to museums, watching television, or listening to the radio—those and other activities that stimulate the mind may cut the risk of Alzheimer's disease.

Day 320

ACTIVATE YOUR HEARING

*He who has an ear, let him hear what the
Spirit says....* —REVELATION 3:22

Ears are designed for hearing. Hearing God's Word and allowing it to settle in and permeate your spirit promotes life. Our Creator, in His infinite wisdom, knows that clean machines work better. Your body's self-healing nature can use ear canals for a detoxification site. I generally see abundant earwax in individuals with compromised digestion, elimination, and toxic eating habits. For instance, individuals who smoke generally have more accumulation of wax than nonsmokers.

CARPAL TUNNEL PAIN

*...and none of the mighty men have found
the use of their hands.* —PSALM 76:5

Do you suffer with carpal tunnel syndrome (CTS)? Try eliminating soda, cookies, and dairy from your snack habit. Drink purified water and eat almonds and veggie sticks as an alternative. Adding pain-relieving flax oil from an organic source, one tablespoon per 100 pounds of body weight along with 150 milligrams of whole food vitamin B6, will promote healing of the inflamed tissues. CTS of both wrists may be precipitated by a misaligned or a decayed neck vertebra and disc.

LIFE WITHOUT BACK PAIN

Why is my pain perpetual and my wound incurable, which refuses to be healed?... —JEREMIAH 15:18

Back pain for long duration caused by food sensitivities versus bone or joint injury miraculously disappears when you delete dairy and citrus and stop smoking cigarettes. Test me on this!

STICKS AND STONES WILL BREAK MY BONES

He guards all his bones; not one of them is broken. —PSALM 34:20

Did you ever break a bone? Fractures can be painful, especially the ones that you cannot support or cast, such as a tailbone or nose. Bones have a rich supply of blood vessels and nerve endings. Regardless of what you do, it takes time for bones to heal and replace themselves. Osteoporosis fracture prevention can be helped with flax oil. Flax oil helps restore hormone function and calcium absorption.

"HE KNOWS OUR FRAME"

For He knows our frame; He remembers that we are dust. —PSALM 103:14

Try "toe raises" to alleviate pain. While sitting in a stationary position with your feet straight forward and flat on the floor, raise your toes 25 times. Then turn your feet inward and repeat the toe raises 25 times. Turn your feet outward and repeat. This will strengthen foot structure, which supports the frame.

BUILDING STRONG BONES

*...And a good report makes the bones
healthy.* —PROVERBS 15:30

When you are under emotional distress,
your body uses more calcium to neutralize the acid environment caused by the
negative emotions. That is why you will see
cold sores or fever blisters on people who are
having higher than normal negative emotional pressure. Your bones need calcium,
protein, and other ingredients to be strong.

PLANTAR FACIITIS—
FOOT PAIN

*From the sole of the foot even to the
head, there is no soundness in it, but the
wounds and bruises and putrefying sores;
they have not been closed or bound up, or
soothed with ointment.* —ISAIAH 1:6

Burning feet are usually caused by poor
or improper fat metabolism precipitated
by a congested liver and a limited intake
of vitamin B, including Choline and Ino-
sitol. Plantar Fasciitis, which is pain along
the tissue on the very bottom of the foot
and heel area, is normally caused by not
enough Omega 3 flax oil consumption, lack
of vitamin B6, low thyroid, and weak adrenals. Thyroid function is needed for calcium
absorption, which calms and relaxes tissues.

LESSONS LEARNED FROM MUMMIES

Now when they had departed, behold, an angel of the Lord appeared to Joseph in a dream, saying "Arise, take the young Child and His mother, flee to Egypt, and stay there until I bring you word...." —MATTHEW 2:13

We have been blessed to learn from studying the remains of Egyptian mummies. They ate a diet much like we do. Low fat, high carbohydrate, grains, and corn residue have been discovered in their stomachs upon dissection. Their blood vessels had scarring similar to individuals today who have high blood pressure. Learn from the past. Increase flax oil consumption necessary to relieve pain and blood vessel inflammation.

She Was Bent Over

And He laid His hands on her, and immediately she was made straight, and glorified God. —Luke 13:13

Do you know the most common causes of relentless pain? Cigarette smoking, sugar, soda, citrus, white potatoes, and peanut butter. There may be others. What you put in your mouth becomes you. These items may be pain initiators, and cigarettes always slow the healing process. Stop and think before you eat: Does this food promote or subtract from my health bottom line?

THE RIDDLE OF RIGHT KNEE PAIN

Therefore strengthen the hands which hang down, and the feeble knees. —HEBREWS 12:12

Knee pain can be baffling. Carrying more weight on one foot due to trunk alignment imbalance stresses the knees. Pain on the inside of the knee can be decay or cartilage and ligament tearing. General knee cap pain may be bursitis. Daily taking flax oil (one tablespoon per 100 pounds of body weight), 150 milligrams of B6, and organic apple cider vinegar relieves bursitis.

Day 330

BE ALL YOU CAN BE

Jesus came to give us life to the fullest, to live in abundance. We are the builders of God's Kingdom on the earth. Chronic, repetitive stress can be annoying and, in fact, disabling. It is challenging to give 100 percent if you don't feel 100 percent. I encourage eating alfalfa sprouts and tablets as a source of sodium. You need sodium to have pliable muscles and tissues.

STAY CONNECTED TO THE SOURCE

Abide in Me, and I in you. As the branch cannot bear fruit by itself, unless it abides in the vine, neither can you, unless you abide in Me. —JOHN 15:4

We all need to be connected to the vine—Jesus. Without Jesus, we can do nothing. You can become disconnected from the source by trauma or injury. When a vertebra moves and compresses a nerve, whatever tissue the nerve innervated will stop working at 100 percent. Have you tried a variety of remedies and there is little to no improvement in your condition? Then it is time to be checked for subluxation by a skilled natural spinal specialist.

FEET WERE MADE TO WALK

Ponder the path of your feet, and let all your ways be established. —PROVERBS 4:26

Do you know—this may sound far-fetched—that you can get indigestion because of a misaligned foot bone? Yes. I have manually corrected a subluxated foot bone called the talus. The foot bone is connected to the ankle bone, which is connected to the knee, hip, and pelvis. The lumbar spine affects the muscles associated with hiatal hernia. Correcting the foot position impacts the entire body.

SUBLUXATION

*These things I have spoken to you,
that in Me you may have peace. In
the world you will have tribulation*
[thlipsis]; *but be of good cheer, I have
overcome the world.* —JOHN 16:33

Look at your full posture today. Close your eyes, tilt your head, back and forth. Open them. Look in the mirror. Now does you head shift? Is your neck centered and shoulders level? Have someone take a side posture view with a digital camera; your ear should be perpendicular to your shoulder. Correcting subluxation and strengthening and improving posture will result in an improved level of optimal health. Seek a natural spinal adjuster.

What's in Front of Your Eyes?

And I, Daniel, alone saw the vision,
for the men who were with me did not
see the vision.... —Daniel 10:7

Elijah saw in the spirit what his servant could not see until he prayed for his eyes to be opened. Daniel, Jacob, and Paul saw a vision. My prayer is for you to have your eyes opened for your health's sake. The Power who made the body—our heavenly Father—breathed life into us to heal the body.

JOINTS

And not holding fast to the Head, from whom all the body [is] *nourished and knit together by joints and ligaments....* —COLOSSIANS 2:19

Sulfur and other minerals and elements are used by the body for joint strength. Sulfur helps make collagen a critical factor for joint, skin, muscle, and ligament strength. Excellent sources of sulfur include eggs, onion, garlic, radishes, and cabbage. A heavy phlegm in the throat is a body signal of a sulfur deficiency.

Personal Evolution

*For everyone who partakes only of milk is
unskilled in the word of righteousness, for he
is a babe. But solid food belongs to those who
are of full age, that is, those who by reason
of use have their senses exercised to discern
both good and evil.* —Hebrews 5:13-14

Achieving new levels of health takes
courage in a culture where billions of
prescriptions are consumed. Peak performance requires energy and the capacity to
change or else you will continue in the same
downward spiral of poor health. Are you on
antidepressants? Focus on increasing flax oil,
one tablespoon per 100 pounds body weight.
Add more protein, along with 150 milligrams of B6 a day for three months. Do you
suffer with constipation? Increase your water
consumption and raw vegetables.

ADDRESSING CHRONIC HEALTH ISSUES

If you constantly deal with chronic sinus problems, eliminate dairy and peanut butter. Shoulder pain can be corrected by eliminating citrus. Do you have morning headaches? Cease eating sweet fruit or sweet snacks before bed. Chocolate cravings? Eat mixed green salads daily. To curb your desire for dairy, try focusing on olive and flax oil for fat along with sesame seeds for calcium and protein.

HEALTHY WEIGHT LOSS

A re you struggling to lose weight? Drink more water and minimize your sweets. Sweets increase insulin. You will have challenges losing weight with elevated insulin. Leg cramps while sleeping can be eliminated by adding sesame seeds and almonds to your diet.

TENNIS ELBOW

*He has shown strength with
His arm....* —LUKE 1:51

Arm pain, especially elbow pain, prevents
even the basic of human functions.
Elbow pain on the outside aspect is seen in
motions of twisting the arm and hand, as
in hitting a tennis ball. For chronic pain,
supplement your diet with an anchovy/
sardine based marine oil for three weeks,
taking two teaspoons a day for three weeks;
then take only flax oil with a whole food B6
(150 milligrams daily), and apple cider vinegar, one tablespoon a day.

LIPOSUCTION: NO HEART SAVER

If you're overweight, eat less and exercise more. Liposuction may shed pounds—but not risk. It doesn't make you take in fewer calories than you burn. Another possibility? Although it removes fat cells that are subcutaneous (just under the skin), liposuction doesn't shrink fat cells or remove the fat that's deeper in the abdomen, liver, and muscles.

RESTFUL, PEACEFUL SLEEP

Your body repairs itself during restful, peaceful sleep. Plan your daily routine; manage your time in such a way that you are in bed before midnight. Avoid activities that are not productive. Procrastination steals sleep time. Have a sleep schedule that is consistent with your meal planning, exercise, and quiet time.

DEEP SLEEP

And the Lord God caused a deep sleep to fall
on Adam, and he slept.... —GENESIS 2:21

The best sleep is a deep, God-sleep. Adam and Saul both were in a deep sleep, Adam for a rib to be removed to create woman and Saul for David's safety. Sleep is when your body has the opportunity to do all the repairs. People today with the rush of life, stress, and anxiety generally do not get the sleep they need.

Restful Sleep

I encourage patients to exercise during the day, if possible. Exercise promotes movement and cleansing of fluids and toxins. Endorphins released during exercise create an atmosphere of calmness. Calcium citrate and lactate help people fall asleep and prevent leg cramps at night. Turkey and tuna have tryptophan, which is a sleep precursor. Eat sesame seeds, calcium lactate, or citrate with a turkey or tuna dinner as sources of calcium and tryptophan to promote initial sleep drowsiness.

LAUGHTER—GOD'S HEART MEDICINE

...we were like those who dream. Then our mouth was filled with laughter, and our tongue with singing.... —PSALM 126:1-2

Do you take time to laugh? Laughter is God's medicine for the heart. Laughter relaxes blood vessels boosting blood flow. Life is in the blood. It carries essential nutrients and oxygen to tissue cells. When you laugh, reactions in the body are prompted by a release of nitric oxide, which relaxes blood vessels much like endorphins released during exercise. When you laugh, you also have less wear on your joints.

TISSUE REPAIRS OCCUR DURING SLEEP

...Both the chariot and horse were cast into a dead sleep. —PSALM 76:6

Restful, peaceful sleep without interruption of natural body function is essential to promote organ and tissue revitalization. Poor calcium utilization and resulting deficiencies prevent the initial calmness to achieve initial sleep.

Day 346

LEG CRAMPS AND CALCIUM

Leg cramping while lying down at night is a common body signal suggesting a need for calcium. Sesame seeds, almonds, and mixed greens added to your diet would be a good start as they are easily assimilated by the body. If you are currently taking an over-the-counter calcium supplement and have night leg cramps, try another product with calcium citrate or lactate. Avoid digestive aid calcium products that contain calcium carbonate; they are more difficult to absorb.

DEPRESSION FREEDOM

*Anxiety in the heart of man causes
depression, but a good word makes
it glad.* —PROVERBS 12:25

Feeding on the Word of God fills a void;
without the Word, people are empty. A
leading cause of depression is a lack of quality nutrients in the diet. An organic source
of Omega 3 flax oil (one tablespoon per day
per 100 pounds body weight) promotes the
formation of DHA needed for brain health.
Whole food B vitamins and minerals create
an environment for emotional stability.

REDUCING DEPRESSION

Eliminate sugar from your life. Sugar robs the body of substances needed to complete the formation of fat for brain activity. Human-made trans fat or partially and hydrogenated fats sabotage every cell reaction and can lead to emotional imbalance, including ADHD. Exercise promotes "feel good" endorphin production in the body, which reduces anxiety.

COMBATING DEPRESSION

For emotional stability take either two teaspoons of an anchovy/sardine-sourced marine oil or one tablespoon of flax oil per 100 pounds of body weight. An Essential Fatty Acid or EFA blood spot test is a wise test allowing you to create the proper fat/oil supplementation protocol.

SWEET SLEEP

After this I awoke and looked around, and my sleep was sweet to me. —JEREMIAH 31:26

Elevated tissue copper levels may keep your brain racing even if your body is exhausted. Increasing calcium-rich food sources (like sesame seeds, almonds, and mixed greens) helps. Low calcium may prevent drowsiness. Consuming turkey and tuna increases natural sources of tryptophan, a necessary ingredient for sleep. Minimize caffeinated products, including the obvious coffee and tea, but also chocolate. You need optimal liver function to process caffeine.

THE LAMP OF YOUR BODY

The lamp of the body is the eye. If therefore your eye is good, your whole body will be full of light. —MATTHEW 6:22

Light penetrates to the back of the eye. You actually see with your brain through the two "video cams," or your eyes. Jesus healed the blind. You can be physically and spiritually blind since the natural person does not receive the things of the Spirit of God (see 1 Cor. 2:14). Your ability to receive sunlight is affected by your mineral level consumption.

EAT WHOLE FOODS

Does bright light bother your eyes? Eat less sugar and eat more cucumbers. Trouble driving at night? Eat more carrots. Are your eyes dry? Try iodine first for three months and potassium if that does not help. Are cataracts blurring your vision? Have your calcium and phosphorus level checked by your healthcare provider. The ratio should be ten parts calcium to four parts phosphorous. An imbalance with excessive calcium may result in a cloudy lens. We encourage eating grains and protein to lower the calcium. Eat whole foods.

REST IN THE LORD

*Rest in the Lord, and wait patiently
for Him....* —PSALM 37:7

God, yes God, rested on the seventh day. He created the entire universe; then He rested. Wow! If God rested, that is definitely a mandate for us to rest. A couple of tips: Stress and anxiety interrupt a normal pattern of sleep. If you have difficulty achieving sleep, try shutting off the television and stop reading the news. Play soothing instrumental praise and worship music to calm the spirit. Let your brain have a break from noise as it settles down for the evening.

Day 354

A FULL NIGHT OF SLEEP

Do you wake up two hours after you fall asleep? Take a whole food B vitamin before you lay your head down. I encourage flat or low pillows so your head is not raised but horizontal to the bed. Cover the alarm, VCR, and TV lights in your room. They disrupt deep sleep. Minimize caffeine before bed. Do you or your spouse snore? Put a wedge of lemon in hot water and sip on it. Then eat the lemon. Waking up hungry is a positive body signal that your body is creating growth hormone—which suggests healing is occurring.

WWJD?

Economics has a lot to do with health. The industry, affected by decisions on health research, will complain and minimize reports that negatively affect them. Heart disease, cancer, Alzheimer's, digestive distress, and depression are affected by the politics of health. The Word says to eat food from plants that yield seed, not genetically-modified food. Therefore, eat certified organic food. Avoid human-made foods, including human-made substitutes for sugar and fat. Eat the real thing.

Day 356

Time Well Spent

*And the Lord said to [Ananias], "Arise and go to the street called Straight, and inquire at the house of Judas for one called Saul of Tarsus, for behold, he is praying." —*Acts 9:11

It's been said that you will be the exact same person in five years, except for two events that occur in your life—the people you meet and the books you read. Read books that promote spiritual or physical life. Avoid books that only entertain or amuse you. Pray for new people to come into your fellowship circle. Read one new book this month. Cultivate one new solid relationship with someone this year.

The Cheerful Giver

So let each one give as he purposes in his heart, not grudgingly or of necessity; for God loves a cheerful giver. —Second Corinthians 9:7

Now hear me on this. Position your life to give, help, and teach. No doubt you've heard the saying: Give a man a fish; feed a man for a day. Teach a man to fish; feed him for a lifetime. It's true that life skills are necessary for a happy, successful life. Giving is God's economy. Help those in need. Be a blessing to someone anonymously now, and you will be rewarded in Heaven later.

Day 358

STOOL SECRETS

*"...Are you thus without understanding also? Do you not perceive that whatever enters a man from the outside cannot defile him, because it does not enter his heart but his stomach, and **is eliminated, thus purifying** all foods?"* —MARK 7:18-19.

Fiber increases the passage of the food. You don't get adequate fiber from white bread, doughnuts, fries, and pastries. Regular consistent fiber food, especially apples, are good for the colon. Fiber gently scrapes the colon walls. Psyllium tends to absorb too much water, dehydrating the colon. Flax fiber and powder is a better choice. Diarrhea may be a sign of lactose issues or even toxicity.

Baths and Sleep

A hot bath before bedtime raises the body's temperature, and the subsequent cooling may trigger sleep. A hot bath with mineral salts will help calm the tissues and is an excellent source of minerals. Avoid toxic-sourced bubble bath compounds.

STAY STRONG

*So the Lord said, "Simon, Simon! Indeed, Satan has asked for you, that he may sift you as wheat. But I have prayed for you, that your faith should not fail; and when you have returned to Me, **strengthen your brethren**."* —LUKE 22:31-32

Being strong physically is necessary to staying strong spiritually. It is much more of a challenge to do the Lord's work when you are physically exhausted. Spend time with your family and friends. Minimize the time you are entertained by media. Initiating this lifestyle promotes spiritual and physical strength. "Early to bed, early to rise, makes a man healthy, wealthy, and wise." —Benjamin Franklin

SEASONED WITH SALT

Salt enhances the taste of food by drawing out the "au jus" from entrees. I encourage using natural Celtic Sea Salt; it has not been colored or chlorinated. Chlorine is often used by commercial brands to whiten their salt product. Aluminum, a known toxin when in abundance on neuron structures, and dextrose, a sugar, have been used as anticaking factors.

ARISE AND SHINE

Arise, shine; for your light has come!
And the glory of the Lord is risen
upon you. —ISAIAH 60:1

To quote Benjamin Franklin again, "Early to bed, early to rise, makes a man healthy, wealthy, and wise." The hours you sleep before midnight are critical for optimal health. The adrenal gland, which is located on top of your kidneys, makes cortisone. When you go to bed late, your adrenal glands have to work harder. The adrenals will wear out over time. You may have pain and belly fat due to always having to get your "second wind."

HEALTHY SLEEP

Focus on being in bed by ten. Exercise during the day will help you be in a state to fall asleep. Turkey is an excellent source of tryptophan needed to make a hormone for sleep. Minimize caffeine after dinner. Caffeine is found in chocolate, sodas, and some painkillers. Some teas even have more caffeine than coffee. Trouble falling asleep will improve by eating calcium-rich sesame seeds. You will get the best deep sleep when all light sources are eliminated.

WATCH WHAT YOU TOUCH

When the army goes out against your enemies, then keep yourself from every wicked thing....But it shall be, when evening comes, that he shall wash with water.... —DEUTERONOMY 23:9,11

Wash your hands, and watch what you put in your mouth. Only eat cooked food, not burnt, with no undercooked "au jus" or flesh present. Do not let children play in uncovered sandboxes. Be mindful of outside cats that eat mice. Do not eat sushi. If you have pain in your body after eating sushi, you need to be tested for parasites.

BE A BLESSING EVERY DAY!

*And He led them out as far as Bethany,
and He lifted up His hands and
blessed them.* —LUKE 24:50

I have heard it preached that it is grander to receive blessings than it is to need a miracle. I suggest you look for blessings in your life. If you do not expect or look for them, you may not find them. I have patients tell me every day how blessed they have been to learn that they can have an impact on their own lives. I am glad that you finished the book, and pray that you pass on what you have learned. If I don't see you here on earth...look for me in Heaven.

ABOUT DR. BOB DEMARIA

Dr. Bob DeMaria is an experienced natural healthcare provider. He has focused his career on helping patients with drugless therapeutic protocols. Dr. Bob has a degree in Human Biology, specialties in Spinal Engineering and Natural Orthopedic Treatment. He graduated cum laude and the valedictorian of his class. He practices clinically as a Chiropractor (DC). Dr. Bob continually pursues advanced educational opportunities and is currently studying to earn a Natural Health Doctor (NHD) degree.

Dr. Bob co-hosts a TV program with Deb, his wife of over thirty-five years. He has been a college instructor, team physician, business health consultant, and post-graduate trainer in the legal and health fields. He has written six other books, which are available at www.druglessdoctor.com. Dr. Bob also has several workshop audio series including, "Dr. Bob's Top 10 Tips for Wellness."

Dr. Bob is an international speaker, has served as an expert witness, and has been in an active practice since 1978. He gave his life to the Lord in 1987. He and his wife, Debbie, appreciate the prayers of all who read this book. They have two sons, Dominic and Anthony. A portion of the proceeds from this book will be used to financially support Bethany Blessing Ministry.

Dr. DeMaria is available on a limited basis to speak at your next corporate event or convention. His energetic speaking style will inspire, educate, and motivate your employees to greater levels of health, wealth, and personal confidence. Dr. Bob's enthusiasm for life is contagious!

Contact information:
Phone: 1-888-922-5672
Fax: 440-323-1566
Email: drbobdemaria@gmail.com

BOOKS BY DR. ROBERT DEMARIA

Dr. Bob's Drugless Guide to Detoxification

This may be the most toxic time in history. Daily headlines report the negative conditions of our water, food, and air. The "green movement" is popularly creating a mindset to secure a safer, cleaner environment, but little is said about the circumstances our bodies have to contend with. This book is a logical plan that establishes true wellness in your body from the inside out. Dr. Bob shares clinically proven, time-tested protocols that can be followed in the comfort of your own home—no need to travel to expensive clinics or follow strict and stressful diet plans. You will learn what to purchase at your own grocery store to maintain a healthy body, be empowered to make wise choices and not be dependent on medications, avert possible surgical intervention to remove an exhausted dysfunctional organ, and learn what to eat and what to avoid to create an optimally functioning cellular environment!

Dr. Bob's Guide to Stop ADHD in 18 Days

A Drugless Family Guide to Optimal Health

Anyone can successfully overcome ADHD and hyperactivity without drugs. This book details how to get your children and family off medications and detrimental junk foods filled with trans fatty acids, dairy products, sugar, and preservatives, so that they can have optimal, natural health. This is a simple, effective step-by-step plan that includes adding flax oil and modifying your diet and vitamin/mineral intake. The protocol will improve your nervous system function, and help you overcome behavioral and learning problems. It will improve insomnia, mood swings, and irritability. The result will be your body healing itself naturally. Participants in the pilot program saw improvement in only 18 days. NATURALLY!

Dr. Bob's Drugless Guide to Balancing Female Hormones

The time tested information in this book is designed to create a state of optimal health in the female hormonal system. Dr. Bob's insight into cell function empower readers to make wise choices designed to nourish and detoxify the body with items that can be easily incorporated in a day-to-day routine. You will learn that a clear and clean lymphatic system is important and that a functioning liver is vital for balance. The role of nutrients like iodine and proper oil help create the foundation needed to progress into hormonal maturity without annoying body signals. You will be exposed to the procedures that Dr. Bob has used to transition his patients into feeling great without medication.

Dr. Bob & Debbie's Guide to Sex and Romance

This book is a collection of personal and clinically based evidence including protocols applied and successfully used from Dr. Bob's healthcare practice. Dr. Bob and Debbie also share their common sense experience from 40 years of their personal relationship and over 30 years of marriage. You will gain from the insight they have gleaned from their involvement and observations discovered while being in natural health since 1978. The DeMaria's have watched the decline of the overall personal health of the new patients presented to the clinic and discuss the restoration of those individuals' overall health. Dr. Bob linked the associated deterioration of sexual desire and whole body dysfunction with patients having chronic health challenges.

Dr. Bob's Men's Health—The Basics

This book is for men who want simple, honest answers to their basic health questions. In today's culture women tend to make the majority of the healthcare decisions for their families—while men tend to avoid seeking care, oftentimes until the pain and discomfort caused by the conditions they have suffered with are beyond their ability to cope. Dr. Bob's extensive experience as a healthcare provider, without the use of prescription medication, has provided him with a unique ability to understand and relay logical solutions in an easy-to-follow format. In this book, Dr. Bob reveals important, little known facts on the more common conditions men contend with: heart disease, cancer, cholesterol, sexual dysfunction, and pain. You will learn the basics which will propel you to levels of optimal health, without the use of prescription medication.

Dr. Bob's Trans Fat Survival Guide
Why No Fat, Low Fat, Trans Fat is KILLING YOU!

This book explains the dangers of trans fat, commonly called hydrogenated and partially hydrogenated fat, as well as how to recognize it in everyday food by properly reading nutritional labels. Along with trans fat, you will learn the different types of fats, which ones are beneficial, and which ones should be used for cooking, baking, or eating. Not to leave the reader hanging with questions on how to eliminate dangerous fats and take on a healthier approach to life, there are several sections dealing with how to make those changes, transitioning healthier foods into their eating plan. This book will encourage and empower you to make better choices and learn to live an optimal and healthy life.